Stretching & HOGUSHI Massage

To prevent injuries and ease pain

by Saburo Ishii

President of Family Yoga
Tokyo, Japan

Published by:

Zen Central
PO Box 5046
West End Qld 4101
Australia
www.zencentral.com.au

First English Edition, October 2011

ISBN 978-0-646-56499-9

Printed by Paradigm Print Media, Brisbane, Australia.

Saburo Ishii

Saburo Ishii was born in Tokyo in 1944. He has been researching Zen, Buddhist prayers, sleep improvement methods, fasting, Soutaihou (Natural Movement) and Hatha yoga for more than 40 years.

He started studying Oki Yoga under Masahiro Oki, the founder of Oki Yoga, in 1977. Soon after, he and his wife Hisae Ishii, established the Family Yoga School in Kanda, Tokyo. For more than 30 years he's been teaching yoga and fasting at classes, workshops and retreats.

As well as teaching in Japan, he's also taught in Taiwan, Brazil, Australia and America, building networks around the world. He is an advisor to Taiwan Oki-do Yoga. He's also written *Karadanikiku Yoga* (published in Japanese by Gendaishorin).

Website: www.family-yoga.jp

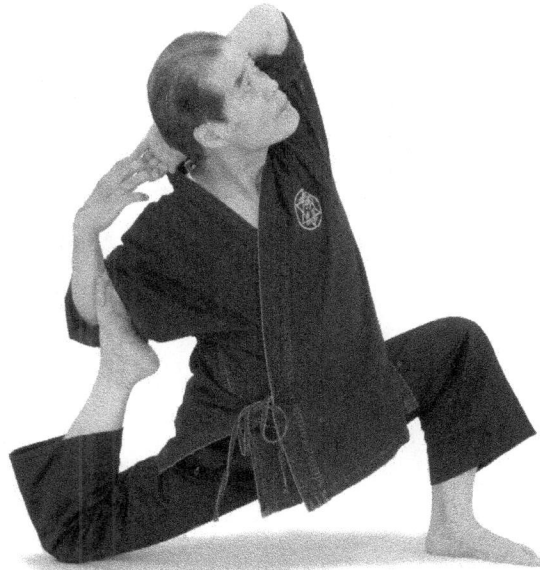

Foreword

To be centred; spiritually, intellectually and personally all depends upon a sound somatic practice. Too easily we forget that our social, intellectual and professional lives are grounded in our bodies and in its function. Even this statement is a misconception as it is not 'our bodies' but the physical foundation of self, which underpins life. Our professional, social and family life depends on a strong awareness of somatic well-being.

Master Ishii has been a lifelong practitioner of Zen, yoga and mental awareness with over 40 years experience. He teaches not only in Japan but also in Taiwan, Australia, Brazil as well as creating networks in many other countries. He is a gifted teacher. Master Ishii's simple yet elegant approach to managing the body-mind is of enormous benefit to all. This approach can be practised by everyone and requires a fine attention to oneself. The way is easy but profound in effect. This is truly 'teaching with the heart' and I recommend this valuable book with all its wisdom.

Daniel Weber PhD; MSc

Preface

I decided to write this book to introduce HOGUSHI (pronounced HOG SHE) Massage to a broader audience. I believe it has a wide range of benefits; from preventing sports and work related injuries, to facilitating a lighter and more energised daily life.

It is based on my experiences, and is for people who have pain in their daily life due to body stiffness, sporting injuries and so on. I want to let them know that they might be more comfortable by applying HOGUSHI Massage for the body and mind.

For people who have knee pain when they go up and down stairs, applying Hips HOGUSHI Massage will reduce their pain. Sports participants can enhance their performance and prevent injury by taking enough time for warm ups with HOGUSHI Massage and stretching.

HOGUSHI Massage is effective for health care

By releasing muscle stiffness, people generally feel much better from the resulting increase in the blood and lymph flow and stabilised body temperature. This tends to make them feel lighter, more energised and able to work more efficiently. They are also able to maintain their physical condition and alleviate fatigue quickly, which helps to prevent injuries and create a fresh start for the next day. With this good body maintenance program, sports skills improve faster and people can continue to play their favourite sport with joy.

As a child, I was often made fun of due to my short stature. I felt resentment towards these people, which I now realise created conflict within myself. Through yoga I learnt how to open the mind.

By releasing the body and mind, it's easier to have a relaxed life. I have been practising yoga for more than 40 years and know that I have been able to experience an easier and more fulfilling life because of it.

I could not be happier if you too can come to feel that it supports your health and wellbeing and is able to provide you with a spiritually rich and satisfying life along with a flexible body.

HOGUSHI Massage is accepted internationally because it works!

Each year, I am invited by yoga groups to hold workshops in Taiwan and Australia and I have been teaching them HOGUSHI Massage.

When teaching in Australia, I saw that previous students were using HOGUSHI Massage before the workshop. I assumed they were using what was taught several years ago because it was helpful to them.

They had realised that the techniques taught were beneficial and made it easier to practise some yoga poses. I was very pleased to witness that HOGUSHI Massage is acknowledged and used overseas as well as in Japan.

I would like to take this opportunity to thank the Oki-do Master, President Haku and his wife Mrs Haku, both of whom taught and guided me in how to be aware of the heart, and hence, to follow and live from the heart.

Additionally, Mr Mikihito Nagai and Mr Takao Kikuike gave me the opportunity to research Shiatsu and Sotai and that helped greatly to expand my ideas and techniques.

Also, I appreciate all of the students who are practicing HOGUSHI Massage and have provided evidence that it works effectively.

I also take this opportunity to thank the models; Ms Hirona Hisako and Ms Masami Otsubo, the illustrator- Ms Chika Honyashiki, my Japanese publisher- Ms Kobayashi, Ms Sekiguchi and Mr Asao from Gendaishorin, the assistant, Ms Miharu Sakurai, for publishing this book and understanding my unreasonable demands, all of which have been a new endeavour for HOGUSHI Massage. And last but not least, a special thanks to my wife, Hisae Ishii, who did the proof reading many times.

For the first edition in English, I would like to thank Takatoyo Yamamoto for the original translation from Japanese to English. Also, a big thanks to Peter Masters for overseeing the project from start to finish along with editing and proof reading. I'd like to thank Linden Brooks and Barbara Rooke for their extensive editing and proof reading. Also to thank Angela Hammond for her work on the design and layout of the book. And a special thankyou to Masako Kunino for her support and friendship over many years.

Saburo Ishii
President of Family Yoga
Tokyo, Japan
October 2011

Stretching and HOGUSHI Massage

To prevent injuries and ease pain

Many people play sport for health benefits and for fun. Regrettably, it is often the case that many people have knee, elbow and lower back trouble.

For instance, tennis players can develop tennis elbow and golfers, back pain. Some people pull muscles while doing cardiovascular exercise at gyms. Even in yoga classes, people can injure themselves by incorrect performance of complicated poses, if they are not properly primed to apply them.

A lot of professional athletes underestimate the consequences of minor pains and continue performing. Under such conditions it can be difficult to improve their skills and gain better results.

It is counter-productive to be injured while playing sports, when the purpose is predominantly for health care. However, a lot of people keep playing, even with their aches and pain, as they believe in the concept of, 'no pain, no gain'.

HOGUSHI Massage has been created through personal experience

My height is only 155cm. I was a boxer and long distance runner as a student. I thought these sports would be no trouble for someone with short stature such as myself. After graduation, I worked for nearly ten years in the transport industry to help my father. I regularly carried goods of 40 to 50kg with repetitive movements that tightened my physique. I eventually developed a toned, muscular and stiff body.

After building my body like this, I started yoga, which requires flexibility. It wasn't that easy to make my body softer. To manage this I needed to do something extra such as HOGUSHI Massage.

When I was younger, I had practised yoga with some pain when holding advanced poses. As a result, I became debilitated and was unable to go up and down stairs without holding the handrails. Occasionally, I injured my knees and neck and was not able to turn properly.

At one point, I dislocated my left shoulder and needed to visit an osteopath. My shoulder and arm were immobile due to the pain from the muscles around the area becoming stiff and inflexible.

I worked out through this experience that, although a dislocated and/or broken part of the body should not be moved, the muscles around it should be utilised.

Many people see doctors when they have pain, but as it is often only the symptoms being treated, it will not always result in a pain-free outcome.

In the period when I practised yoga with pain, I reached a certain point where I needed to find a way to ease the discomfort to continue with my practice.

First, I thought about how to ease the pain around the shoulder blades and experimentally applied several techniques. I found that not only was the pain reduced, but also physical fatigue was easily removed.

Next, I applied these techniques to the legs and found it worked well. I progressed to the abdomen, and so on, and after many years have developed what has become my HOGUSHI Massage for the whole body. 'Hogosu' literally means 'slacken the tension' in Japanese. It is my pleasure to pass on the techniques and practice of this life-enhancing massage.

DISCLAIMER

You should consult your doctor or other health adviser before doing any of the poses or exercises in this book if you have a medical condition or injury. Always disclose any medical condition or injury to your yoga teacher. Mild soreness may be experienced after yoga or other exercise; if it persists for more than 2-3 days, consult your health adviser. The author and publisher have taken care in preparing this book but accept no liability for injury or loss resulting from following its contents.

Contents

Part 4: HOGUSHI Massage for your heart 85

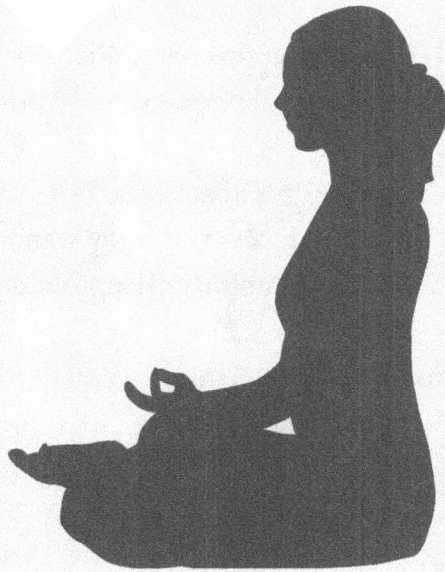

Yoga is generally thought to be good for your health but for some people it can also be damaging.

Many yoga instructors will at times only demonstrate one side of a pose to their students, skipping the other side in order to observe and attend to the whole class. Missing part of the whole movement within the pose can contribute to uneven body alignment.

In general, males are less flexible than females and take longer to gain sustained flexibility. However, males tend to compare their progress with others and push themselves harder for progress, even with evident pain. They often have concepts or attitudes like; "I should be able to do this as well as others" or "I shouldn't be beaten by women".

Some students hold poses with pain and quite often over stretch in poses in an effort to quickly gain flexibility due to their belief in, 'no pain, no gain'. For example Open Legged Forward Bend. As a result, they tend to end up injuring themselves and have to visit masseurs and manipulative therapists to deal with trouble in the back, hips and legs.

Although you shouldn't keep practising with pain, there are two types to recognise, severe pain and pleasant pain.

You should be able to differentiate which type of pain is present by listening to your body.

Severe pain [sharp, deep] remains after exercise. Pleasant pain [mild, relieving] is decreased after exercise and you feel lighter, energised and content with your effort and results.

Oki-do Yoga, which I have practised for many years, is based on the "Teaching of the Heart". In essence, it means 'to do whatever your body wants'. For example, a stooped person may feel invigorated when he stretches himself lengthwise by raising his arms to the sky.

Feeling a "pleasant state of mind" is a confirmation of the "Teaching of the heart".

"Teaching of the heart" never lies. You can confirm it at the time when you recognise a sense of great satisfaction and a calm mind.

In contrast, your body objects when you have severe pain. Under these conditions, it is just a matter of time before you severely damage yourself unless you stop the exercise.

In yoga, you can gradually damage your health if you are continuing with evident pain.

Unlike an instant injury, as in an accident or as caused in some hard sports, it tends to take longer to realise that you have an injured condition.

In the yoga practised in India, there is no concept of callisthenics, as all movements are considered continuous or interconnected in yoga poses. [Callisthenics – simple gymnastic exercises to develop muscle tone and improve general fitness]

The Oki-do Yoga Master I studied with valued callisthenics and ancillary exercises in order to release tightness and increase mobility.

Therefore, I believe, Oki-do Yoga prevents us from severe injuries.

No matter which yoga style people follow, real yogis pay attention to their body condition and, through awareness, tend to find anomalies within themselves. In contrast, this attention and awareness would be difficult for people who do yoga only as a physical sport or as just an exercise regime.

It is detrimental to pursue activities without fundamental physical strength and warming up.

It is important to have fundamental physical strength to play any sports. In order to do so, it is necessary to gain some muscle conditioning and get yourself into good physical shape. Many people however, particularly adults, tend to skip this aspect of the process. It is considered bothersome and people go straight to competitive or game style practice.

There are many cases where people skip thorough warming up before matches. Without warming up with exercises such as HOGUSHI Massage or muscle development training, people can end up causing injuries.

For example, some social volleyball teams spend a period of time practising ball spikes and game strategies, without warm ups or muscle development for optimum physical shape. As a consequence, they can end up with injuries to the shoulders and elbows.

In aerobic classes at gym, instructors tend to make warming up short, due to limited class time and the demands of members. They want to maximise the time dedicated to cardiovascular training and underestimate the importance of warming up.

At youth sports clubs, young people get easily bored with lots of repetitive, fundamental training. They consider running, sit-ups and collecting balls as chores. They just want to play the sport. The profit making clubs need to attract more people, so they tend to offer what members demand, such as skills training instead of foundation training.

It is similar at schools. When visiting a junior high school as a member of the PTA, I noticed warming up was skipped in the physical education class.

Warming up is important as it increases the blood flow and body temperature and helps to avoid preventable injuries. The lack of knowledge of these benefits increases the cases of sports related injuries.

The value of coaches with physiology and sports dynamics knowledge

Sports instructors should know the importance of building fundamental strength and warm ups and teach these principles correctly. However, it seems very few are delivering this.

Employment opportunities at Japanese schools have reduced due to falling birth rates. As a consequence, the number of aged teachers is increasing. Inexperienced teachers often take the supervising role for school teams due to the lack of sports trained coaches.

In regional youth sports clubs, when an appropriate coach is not available, a volunteer parent who has played the sport before becomes the team coach, in spite of little or no training and experience. Often, a volunteer parent who is available on the competition day can become the temporary team coach.

Professional sports players and experienced athletes empirically sense the importance of building fundamental strength and warming up in their own sports field but they usually have little idea of how to apply their specialised knowledge to other sports, as they lack the theory behind it.

It is often said that managers and coaches encourage their players to follow the same methods they were trained in a couple of decades ago, without current and relevant knowledge. The prospect of injuries in training increases as a result.

According to the annual records in 2005, the number of call outs for the Yokohama City Rescue Squad was 2,773 for sports related events.

In statistics from the Japan Sports Promotion Centre, there were 506 cases of injuries under school management in 2006. Around 50% of the cases occurred during physical education classes, sports club activities and sports events at schools.

This number is just the tip of the iceberg. There would be many unreported cases where people have to see a doctor due to injury after sports events, which would not be counted. There would be less preventable injuries if more warming up and fundamental strength training were incorporated.

Using your body correctly to avoid injury

No matter which sport is being played, the risk of injury and damage can always be reduced by being aware of how to use your body correctly.

Many students have no idea about the importance of some fundamental body mechanisms in sports, for example, "tucking the pelvis in" and "tucking the chin in".

In Tai Chi and Karate, many teachers do not focus on correct alignment in the postures. Students bear unnecessary loads on their bodies and this affects their performance. It affects balance, stability and creates more opportunity for injuries.

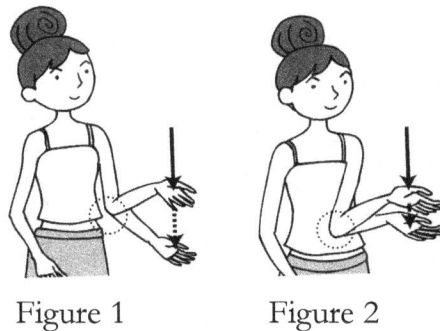

Figure 1   Figure 2

Effective training would be provided if people knew more about body mechanisms such as; "Pulling power is stronger than pushing power in the arms" and "Pushing power is stronger than pulling power in the legs". Another example is the elbows; "it is more stable to tuck the elbow towards the centre of your body", rather than turning it out to the side (see Figures 1 and 2).

"Tucking the elbows toward the centre of the body" is a key to having sustained power in sports.

To illustrate: It is easier for right handed people to tighten a screw clockwise as the right elbow is rotating naturally into the centre of the body. In contrast, it is harder for left handed people to do so, as the left elbow is moving away from the centre of the body.

Like the example mentioned, you can apply natural anatomical mechanisms to your daily life.

Another example is the characteristic of the little finger. When clenching your fist without using the little finger, you will notice that you are not able to get strong power in the grip. Try it again without using the index finger, but focus on using the little finger instead. You will notice that you have more gripping power.

Although it looks smaller than the rest of fingers, the little finger has a great contribution to grip. You can notice more stability in gripping a racket or sword using this mechanism, focusing not on all the fingers, but just the little finger.

Knowledge of body mechanisms can be usefully applied to exercise, sport and health care. It helps to avoid injuries too.

Counter Balance prevents the causes of injury

Repeated stretching of certain parts of the body can lead to some muscles being over stretched. There can be pain and stiffness in an over stretched area. This is due to the body fluids not flowing well and toxins remaining in the area.

By releasing just stretched muscle, body fluids flow better i.e. the blood carries more nutrition and a bolstered lymph system removes toxins. To clarify, we call the action of releasing freshly stretched muscle, "Counter Balance".

Doing a back bend after a forward bend, stretching one side of the body after the other side, closing the legs after opening, are examples. Counter Balance means to stimulate the un-stretched side of a muscle or area of muscle.

After playing a sport, golf for example, it is beneficial to make shadow swings without hitting balls, to twist the body in the opposite direction of the normal swing. For volleyball players, it is beneficial to have shadow ball spikes, using the non-dominant leg to jump and swing the non-dominant arm. By doing Counter Balance, you can avoid uneven body alignment and easily prevent injuries.

To repeat a set of stretching exercises and associated Counter Balances, the muscles are gradually released due to blood and lymph flow improvement, hormone activation and the rise in metabolic body temperature. The effects on the condition of your body are similar to having a hot bath. By the way, it is always good to do 'stretching' after a hot bath as the body is more pliable and can stretch effectively, without adverse pain.

By repeating a set of exercises with Counter Balances, discomfort in your body is gradually reduced and mobility is gradually increased. After playing a sport, muscles recover quickly from stiffness and less time is required for warming up the next day.

Counter Balance is not generally utilised enough. A lot of people do not bother to do stretching. They complain about pain, are unable to gain mobility and overall, show little improvement in their health.

Sports instructors have confidence in their programs as long as stretching, warming up and cooling down time are included, regardless of their quality. When their players complain of pain in a body part or area, they tend to consider that this indicates a weakness in that part of the players' body.

The situation is much the same in ballet and yoga. People suffer preventable lower back pain as they don't do counter balances. An example is someone seeing progress in their flexibility and their ability to do 'the splits'. They eagerly want to continue without delay to gain additional results. This tends to over stretch certain muscles and they end up developing pain in the lower back and inner thigh, as they have not done a counter balance.

People should know that a muscle can be torn by over stretching. Remember: always perform any set of stretching with an associated counter balance. Then you will gain the benefits from better oxygenated blood, lymph drainage and appropriate body temperature.

Uneven movement in sports can create injury

Playing the same sport and using the same muscle groups for a long period of time can cause uneven body alignment through the under use of other muscle groups.

The late Mr Kazuhisa Inao, a star baseball pitcher in the Nishitetsu Lions, had a lump on his torso that had developed through his overly twisted throwing form.

Other professional sports players with similar conditions need to have osteopathic treatment to correct their alignment due to their unnatural body movements.

Soccer players who only kick a ball using the one foot and tennis players who only use one arm can create pains and distortion in their body alignment without counter balance. After using the right foot a lot to kick a soccer ball during practice and matches, the left foot should then be used. In baseball, a right hand batter also needs practice swings using the left hand as a counter balance.

It is very important for people, particularly teenagers in their period of growth, to know the necessity of counter balance to maintain correct body alignment.

Diet with excessive meat and fish can produce body rigidity

One of the causes of a stiff body is related to diet and foods that are eaten.

In recent years, the main food group of many meals has become animal protein such as meat and fish. **Animals need salt in their body to use their muscles** and raise their body temperatures, so, **animal protein and fat naturally contain large amounts of salt**. Additionally, as people usually add salt when cooking, many of us take too much salt in our diet.

When experimenting by having my meals without added salt for several weeks, I could taste the meat and fish by themselves, including the salty flavour within them. Through this experience I realised how much extra salt is normally added to my diet.

Of course we need to take some salt in our diet. We need it to live, as we feel fatigued by a shortage of it. Obviously, we need the right balance of salt intake in our diet.

A vegetarian diet helps to soften your body, but it may lead to poor circulation and fatigue due to excess amounts of potassium and thus less opportunity to build muscles.

Finding balance is important. The numbers and types of human teeth help to indicate the right ratio of food groups in our diet.

Generally, we have a total of 32 teeth: 20 molars, 8 incisors, and 4 cuspids.

Molars, shaped like mortars, are suitable to grind grains. The reason why we have 20 of them is that we are supposed to consume grains as our principal food. Incisors are good for crunching vegetables and the cuspids are for biting and tearing meat.

According to the ratio of our teeth, the ideal food ratio intake would then be Grains: 5, Vegetable: 2, Meat: 1.

However, sports players may need more meat. In that case, they should also increase their vegetable intake as well.

Some people think it is alright to eat a lot of chicken breasts as it is considered to be low in fat and calories, although still a meat. But remember, chicken is still a food that will make the body tighten. Chickens, just like the majority of birds with the ability to fly, have high energy. It is not beneficial if they are eaten a lot.

To cut all intake of animal products for a certain period of time can help people with high blood pressure to improve their condition, as excess salts in the body are expelled. As generally known, babies don't have high blood pressure as it is a 'later life' related illness and developed from unbalanced eating habits.

Blood pressure will not easily drop by reducing salt intake only. To improve the overall constitution, it would be good to cut all animal products such as meats, seafood and dairy products for 6 - 12 months. Then, returning to the previously mentioned diet ratios of Grain: 5, Vegetable: 2, Meat: 1, as this diet would help to maintain normal blood pressure, with an animal product reduced diet.

Your job may contribute to a stiff body and mental stress

There are many typical cases where the body becomes rigid due to occupation. For instance, people who work in the construction or transport industries where lots of hard physical work is required daily.

Mental conditions also have a huge impact on the physical body.

Mental stress at work and home, as well as negative thinking may be contributors to body rigidity too. People who are full of negative emotions like, "I can't do this…" or "I can't stand this…" can make their body tight by internally holding their emotions.

The more negative emotions held, the more effort required to release the stiffness in the body.

Importance of balance: Tightening and Softening

There are two types of sports' groups in terms of 'impact' on the body, one group is tightening and the other is softening.

Karate, marathon running and tennis are examples of body tightening, and of course weight training is one as well.

Examples of softening sports, requiring both muscle strength and flexibility are gymnastics, rhythmic gymnastics and figure skating.

Ultimately, the body with both muscle strength and flexibility is the ideal balance.

There are many cases of professional sports players shortening their careers due to torn muscles and arthritis, as they are only focused on gaining muscle strength through weight training. Without having both muscle strength and flexibility, it is difficult to be a top class player for a long period.

Some professional sportspeople such as golfers Mr Ryo Ishikawa and Tiger Woods and baseball player Mr Ichiro have developed balanced bodies while playing sports that tend to tighten the body. This is reflected in their good competitive results.

Just like top athletes it is still important for everyone to have a balanced body.

Some yoga practitioners mistakenly think flexibility is everything in yoga.

But we also need some muscle strength to live everyday life.

A number of beginner yoga students at my school, usually young women, have very poor strength and are unable to raise their legs from the position of lying on their back.

They may be able to dance well but they lack strength and an overall good health condition.

It is important to have both muscle strength and flexibility, and yoga assists in its ability to contribute to a balanced body.

Part 2:
The reasons why the body needs to be released

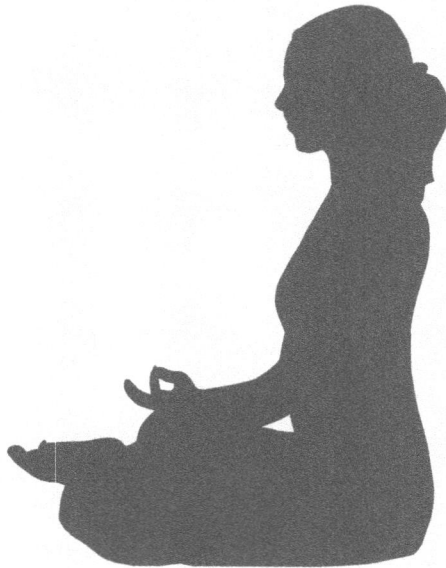

Playing sports for health with HOGUSHI Massage

Callisthenics and HOGUSHI Massage are highly recommended before and after weight training.

The majority of sport players do weight training, regardless of their type of sport. Weight training has a high risk of tightening the body, constricting blood flow and accumulating toxins.

At a sports club I used to attend, a person had a cerebral haemorrhage during a weight training session and was taken by ambulance to hospital and passed away within two days.

A middle-aged woman living near my home did daily walking exercises for her health but damaged her knee one day. As she continued the daily exercise with knee pain the condition got worse and eventually it was necessary to see a doctor. She then had to have an operation to implant artificial joints and ended up being unable to walk without the aid of a walking stick. She did walking exercise for health, but ironically, it didn't work out that way, in fact quite the opposite.

Applying appropriate HOGUSHI Massage before walking or weight training can help to avoid these kinds of extreme cases. It is ideal for people with stiff musculature to do weight training combined with HOGUSHI Massage and include in the diet, foods such as vegetables, some fruit and vinegared foods to soften their muscles.

It is highly recommended before walking to release any hip stiffness and to stimulate the hip joints, particularly for those with weak legs or bad knees. The distance and speed involved would also have to be considered. If you are following the correct training there will be no pain and a general feeling of comfort and contentment.

Diminished pain means better flexibility

The 'sense of pain' increases when the focus is on a painful part of the body.

To demonstrate, when pinched on your right arm, you sense the pain. Then pinch your left arm and focus on the new painful point: you're able to forget the original pain in your right arm. It occurs because your focus shifted from the right arm to the left.

By maintaining your focus upon a pain in the body, it tends to enhance the pain and you are not able to shift your awareness to other areas.

As the adage goes "Love me, love my dog"- when you are fond of someone, you will focus so much on them that you will love their dog as well.

Pain follows the same way, that is; with focus, you feel more pain when thinking about it. Soon, pain appears even before any physical movement.

Therefore, it is possible to reduce pain by not focusing on it and recognising it as a 'signal'. Sensing pain indicates the body has some kind of unusual load on it. Therefore, the signal is to stop the particular motion and release the pain.

Identifying the point of pain and releasing the muscles around it helps to reduce the load and create smoother mobility and correct alignment.

As pain increases by focusing on it, you are able to shift and reduce it by releasing the area. Remember, do not focus on the area that you feel pain, but use it as a signal to make a corrective, right action.

Stretching and HOGUSHI Massage

It is important to do HOGUSHI Massage to reduce pain and prevent injuries. At the same time, stretching is also required. The stretching meant here is not the same type usually used at sport clubs, but yoga poses (asanas).

From the beginning of practice, yoga asanas are for stretching all over the body. Generally, the difference between yoga poses and stretching (as at sports clubs) is that the focus in yoga is on stimulating the target spots by motion and utilising breath.

By focusing on matching the motion and breathing, muscles are stretched smoothly. To practise with 'conscious awareness, breath and motion' in yoga is called "3 Mitsu (Three Mysteries)".

In Japanese, "Mitsu" often means "Secret", but here it means "Difference in awareness among individuals". As there are differences in breathing and consciousness levels, it cannot be taught in a book. It has to be sensed by the individual.

If doing HOGUSHI Massage, why is stretching required? HOGUSHI Massage is for pinpointing and easing pains in the muscles. Stretching is for stimulating the whole body; as a consequence, blood flow is improved, including to areas with pain.

As all body parts are linked, it is not effective to only focus on the area with pain. By releasing an area with pain with HOGUSHI and doing yoga asanas for whole body stretching, your pain will be reduced and the body will become more flexible.

Four principles in HOGUSHI Massage:
Releasing, Shaking, Counter Balance and Repetition

There are four principles in HOGUSHI Massage.

The first principle is releasing the muscles of an area, the second is shaking the area or applying finger pressure (shiatsu), and the third is applying counter balance.

The fourth principal is repetition of the set of releasing, shaking and counter balancing. These are the four principles of HOGUSHI Massage.

In order to ease a muscle part, you need to do a posture (asana). It may help to ease muscles by doing the opposite posture, for example; people with stooped shoulders could bend over backwards. The progress of release depends on the body area. Some parts may be easily released a couple of centimetres while other parts may only be eased five millimetres. The asana definitely progresses further by placing fingers between joints and muscles, shaking the area and applying shiatsu in the right area.

For solid results, when in the appropriate posture, place the fingers into the area to soften. Sometimes the fingers will go straight into the area, perhaps from the side, upwards, deep or shallow. Push and shake the fingers to the limit of comfort in the direction required.

Usually, it is easier to place the fingers between the joints. For example in the elbow, by bending and relaxing the joint the fingers will go deeper. For the shoulders and arms, shaking and using finger pressure along the collarbone is excellent.

After releasing the muscles, apply counter balance as mentioned in Part 1. When doing forward bends, follow with backward bends and so on. By adding a counter balance the contracted muscle areas are released and blood flow is improved.

It is important to repeat a set of HOGUSHI Massage with releasing, shaking, counter balancing and stretching. By releasing and stretching, blood and lymph flow better, helping to remove toxins and increasing the body temperature.

The more repetition, the more pain reduces and mobility increases. Initially, one to three sets may give you some discomfort. Repeat the set several times per body part and you will notice a difference.

Ideally, it is better to do HOGUSHI Massage and stretching twice a day, in the morning and at night. After morning practice, you can minimise the level of fatigue from work and sports throughout the day.

After night practice, you can have a deep and pleasant sleep before awakening the next morning.

Holistic releasing of the body, as all areas are linked

When there is any pain anomaly in the body then not only that particular area is affected, but other parts are usually linked. For example: when wearing tight shoes or even a corn on the sole of the foot, there may be associated lower back or neck pain.

When there is a pain in the body, we unconsciously try to keep balance by adjusting the posture with subtle movements to release the discomfort. Even if we try to get rid of pain in the lower back or neck by a treatment in a specific spot, it won't always work well. It is important to find out the cause of pain to deal with it effectively.

For example, when there is a pain in the hip joint, you need to apply HOGUSHI Massage not only to the hip joint, but also on the hip areas.

Basically, it is effective to apply HOGUSHI Massage to an area of the body and the corresponding area above, eg. if releasing the knees, then also release the hips. See Table 1.

PAIN	The spot to apply HOGUSHI Massage
Ankles	Back of knees
Knees	Hip joints, hips
Lower back	Hips and the surrounding area
Back	Neck, shoulders, hips
Shoulders	Neck, base of head, thoracic vertebra
Fingers and wrists	Elbows, shoulder blades
Neck	Base of head, shoulders

Table 1

Body alignment can be uneven from the way the body is utilised in daily life, i.e. in sitting postures, at work and playing sport.

For areas of the body that are used a lot in daily life, it is useful to apply counter balances as well as HOGUSHI Massage and stretching. For instance, after prolonged work at a desk where the tendency is to bend forward and hunch. Otherwise, the area of discomfort will expand to the surrounding areas.

Examples of stretching and HOGUSHI Massage

Every person has a unique body figure and each individual has their own movement, suppleness, pain tolerance etc. Due to these differences, everybody needs to find the best HOGUSHI Massage and stretching for themselves to gain the benefits of increased flexibility, pain reduction and general well being.

The appropriate HOGUSHI Massage and stretching varies from person to person. Here are some examples.

In the case of tennis players gripping a racquet in one's dominant hand, the weight distribution can be on the right or left leg to maintain balance. When the weight is predominantly on one leg, the same hip has an extra load as well as the lower back, which then throws off the alignment in the pelvic area. Once the pelvis is affected then the spinal cord will also be affected, which gives more loading on the arm and potential injury such as tennis elbow. When such a condition worsens, players are not able to hold anything with their handgrip due to elbow pain.

It is little use to apply HOGUSHI Massage to just the elbow to treat 'tennis elbow'. By releasing the hips, cervical and thoracic areas, lumbar vertebrae and pelvis in conjunction with stretching (yoga poses) the related areas, the pain would be reduced.

So it would be effective for tennis players to practise Bow pose, Plough pose and Hook pose.

Here is another example in relation to typical office workers who sit at a desk for a long time.

When seated for an extended time, people tend to slump down and sit with their back hunched up. Therefore, this position contributes to various conditions: the chest becomes convex, the neck and surrounding muscles tighten and the muscles of the thighs are also shortened and tightened.

The opposite posture is ideal as a counter balance to release muscle tightness. Counteracting the convex shape can be done by selecting poses where the ribs are pushed up, the chest and navel are stuck out, the shoulders are expanded and the muscles around the thighs are opened. The following would be effective to practise: Easing shoulders with Bow pose and Fish pose.

Correcting your body alignment with HOGUSHI Massage at the end of the day

Sleep is very important for our body. We spend 8 hours sleeping per day, that is, one third of our life is spent sleeping.

Why do we need sleep? It is so the body can recover from mental and physical fatigue and it 'resets' us for a fresh start the next day. Whilst asleep the body has a chance to deal with various anomalies, aches and pains. Quite often conditions such as a headache, stomach ache, minor cold etc are spontaneously fixed by a good night's sleep.

While we are awake and conscious, we tend to think with the mind a lot. As a consequence, emotions such as fear or anger are also held within the body. This can create tension. Although we are not conscious when sleeping, it is part of a natural cycle when tired after the day to rest. Part of this unconscious sleep process is to recover from fatigue and fix minor body distortions. Emotional tensions can also be released.

Sleeping postures reflect this. Energetic kids normally toss about a lot while sleeping and they recover from fatigue quickly. When older, people don't move a lot whilst sleeping and it is understood that the ability of spontaneous or natural cures drops with age.

Therefore, HOGUSHI Massage and stretching before sleep helps to reduce physical tension, calms the mind and assists in improving the ability of spontaneous cure whilst asleep.

In order to allow your body to adjust naturally while sleeping, it is important to choose comfortable bedding. The American league baseball player, Mr Ichiro always took his own pillow when on the road in the United States.

I assume he understood the importance of certain practises to have a better sleep.

How amazing that nothing else but just 'sleeping without effort' can fix our body.

The reason perhaps, that you are not able to get up easily in the morning, is that your body maintenance has not been completed yet. HOGUSHI Massage assists with the process of this natural cure, which is unconsciously done whilst sleeping.

Knowing the laws of body movement:

The centre of gravity in your body, its stability, its transfer and its associated movements

By understanding body mechanisms you are able to apply appropriate HOGUSHI Massage and stretching, thus improving skills in sports and avoiding injuries.

In any sport, tucking the pelvis in is important. In Sumo wrestling, an open leg squat posture with slight forward tilt keeps the body stable. This posture naturally activates the inner knees and arches of the feet and creates a solid foundation. There is no strength to push the opponent if the posture is out of balance.

It is important to master a posture with the pelvis tucked in; this is "the Law of Body Stability".

"The Law of Body Stability" is not only important in sports but also in our daily life. One example is moving a heavy object. Bending over from the back and lifting with straight legs can cause back injury or pain. By practising "the Law of Body Stability", in this case, by bending the knees, tucking the pelvis in and keeping the back straight, we can avoid such easily preventable injuries.

When bending the body to the side, you are able to do so smoothly by shifting your weight to the opposite heel; there is then less of a load with the balance shift. By understanding "the Law of Balance Shifting", the risk of injury is reduced.

A typical example where the law of 'balance shifting' is applied in sport is in any ball and batting games, like swinging of racquets or golf clubs. When bending the body over, tuck the pelvis in and slightly loosen the knees to 'shift balance' and maintain a good centre of gravity.

By shifting balance, the range of flexibility and mobility is improved and there will be less stress loads on the body.

There is a famous Japanese radio exercise program, RADIO TAISO, which is widely used in schools, offices and communities. It has quick movements with musical accompaniment. It can also be effective exercise for aged people when the music is arranged in a slow tempo, or without music, as it reduces the impact on the body and allows more time to 'shift the body balance'.

It was mentioned earlier that you should not focus on a particular body part; this is "the Law of Body Linkage". In part 1, it is stated that a posture with an open chest is a key because the pelvis and chin are naturally tucked in, by opening the chest.

By opening the chest and tucking the pelvis in, the chin doesn't go up to the sky unless you force it to. This movement demonstrates that body parts are linked.

When kicking a ball with the right leg, the right arm is naturally pulled back to create balance. We can see how the arm and leg movements are interrelated. When there is some anomaly in the legs, pain can sometimes appear in the neck and/or hand. Additionally, when the pelvis alignment and/or lower back are distorted, you have more chance of a sprain occurring. As our body tries to keep balance using all components, any linked parts have an extra impact overall and have more risk of injury, i.e. unrelated parts can be injured due to the laws discussed.

By knowing the body mechanisms such as "the Law of Body Stability, Balance Shifting and Body Linkage", you are able to effectively improve sports skills and also avoid preventable injuries in daily life.

Using correct methods

You would be injury free if able to use the body correctly.

It is the same for physical training. For example, tucking the chin in is a key for many actions. When a marathon runner slows by raising the chin and shaking the neck, his or her movement goes into a stall. Power is lost in the chin up posture. In training to master the right posture, remembering to tuck the chin in is paramount.

Effective training begins with the basic knowledge of sports physiology. To reiterate; pulling power is stronger than pushing power in the arms and kicking power is stronger than pulling power in the legs.

Try the following with a partner: push your arms forward, towards the person, and note how much power it takes to do so. Now try when pulling their arms towards your body, and note if there is a stronger sense of power.

It is a natural body mechanism that the arms have more strength in pulling. To gain more strength in pushing contradicts the natural mechanisms, and is not effective because the muscle group is not frequently used. Due to this theory, doing a chin up is a better exercise than a push up to improve the pulling power in the arms.

In Karate and Boxing, strong pulling motion supports the movement to punch faster. With the legs, it is effective to train with kicking power. Thigh lifts and squats are useful muscle strengthening exercises for the legs. As the balance of the lower half of the body becomes stable and strengthened running ability also improves.

When training target areas it is good to carefully consider body mechanisms. They can help to avoid ineffective muscle training and the consequent effects of harming internal organ function and adverse blood flow. Overall, it does not help to improve skills and training results without first thinking about the body mechanisms.

Rehabilitation training for aged people

Correct knowledge about the body mechanisms and effective training is beneficial not only for sports but for rehabilitation as well.

During rehabilitation for walking, particularly for aged people, the trainer often asks them to stand from a seated position without due consideration. It is difficult for people with weakened legs to stand up, as the toes and feet are not strong enough to provide adequate support.

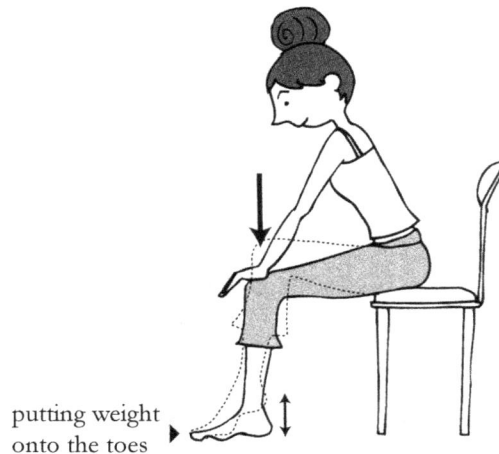

putting weight
onto the toes ▶

Figure 3

They need to build their muscles to stand up through moving the heels up and down while seated, with perhaps some weights on the knees for a while, adding loads onto the toes (see Figure 3). It would seem like torture for them to do walking exercises before building up some physical strength.

People think it is natural that elderly people must have some pains in their body.

It is often heard when aged people are not able to walk properly, "It's no surprise as my grandmother is over 80 years old". But no matter how old we are, pain in the body is just an alert from the body for maintenance.

It is important to remove body pains with appropriate actions to release and relieve.

For example, for those with knee pains: warming the knees and releasing the muscles around the hips would help to reduce pain for aged people, particularly when going up and down stairs.

Releasing internal organs improves blood circulation

The immune system becomes less functional with progressive age. Body temperatures are generally lowered and the ability to generate body heat is diminished. To produce better immune systems, we must build muscular strength. It is important to gain strength in the abdomen, back, arms and legs.

The aim for middle and older aged people is to gain muscular strength for daily life and not to become professional sports players, where they compete with others for progress. It is not necessary to do hundreds of sit-ups at all, just 20 a day is enough. Our physical strength naturally weakens with maturity, so by just adding a little bit of repetition it is more than enough to counter balance the advance of years.

It is better to be sensible with training. Younger people can do 20 or 25 repetitions at once. For older people it's ok to do five times then rest, five times rest etc.

The most important thing is, once again, to apply HOGUSHI Massage before muscle strengthening exercises.

Internal organs can develop bad blood flow over the years, then cells become inactive and back pain can manifest. To improve the immune system, along with gaining muscle strength, we need to create better blood flow in the internal organs.

Ball massage is one of the methods to release the internal organs. Placing a ball like a soccer ball or volleyball under your abdomen and massaging the area by moving up and down, side to side, while controlling your balance with elbows and knees is beneficial (see Figure 4).

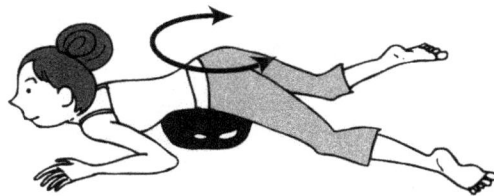

Figure 4

Gaining flexibility with fun

Even though I emphasise that it is important to soften the body, some people respond with negativity such as "It's impossible for me because my body is so stiff", or "it's too late to start for me" etc.

The body will naturally soften with regular and consistent HOGUSHI Massage and stretching (yoga pose/asanas). It can even be done while watching TV or reading a newspaper, eg. open legged seated pose.

The body becomes softer as long as the **practice is completed with a positive sense of joy**, with goals such as:
  − Trying to soften the body little by little   or
  − To exercise for the state of a good mind.

Our bodies are essentially made flexible, as you can see in a baby's movement. With usage over the years our bodies can become stiff and unbalanced. Releasing target areas by 'releasing and shaking' with the fingers between the muscles and joints, greatly improves your flexibility.

The more supple the body, the more pleasure you feel as a result; like a feeling of a refreshing bath, it also encourages you to practise to become even more flexible. Unlike some sports that provide you with continuous pain, a characteristic of HOGUSHI Massage is that it ultimately provides you with pleasure.

The Meaning of Yoga and Yoga Training

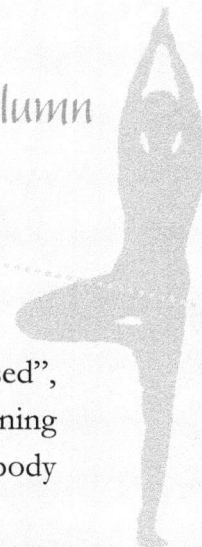

'Yoga' from the Sanskrit definitions means: "to connect to God", "to be harmonised", "to be balanced". Yoga is not just a physical exercise but also a comprehensive training to have a balanced life and includes diet, breathing methods, physical use of the body and ways of thinking.

Maharishi Patanjali systemised yoga training into eight stages in terms of the human mind around the second century B.C. Although it is formed in eight stages, it doesn't mean each stage is a progressive step up, stage by stage. All of the stages are practised simultaneously.

In Oki-do Yoga, which is my basis, the Master added two more stages to make a total of ten stages as follows:

1. **Yama/Niyama:** Readiness
2. **Asana:** Posture
3. **Pranayama:** Breathing Technique and Diet
4. **Pratyahara:** Self-control
5. **Dharana:** Mental Concentration
6. **Dhyana:** Stability
7. **Bhakti:** Do your best and surrender to God
8. **Samadhi:** Unity
9. **Buddhi:** Respect for one's own and others' mind
10. **Prasad:** Real Joy

The difference between Maharishi Patanjali's eight limbs of yoga and Oki-do's is:

– No. 7 was added. Bhakti or Faith means to candidly accept yourself and others' life and the teachings of the body and heart.

Bhakti is not used in the devotional sense but in the sense that it opens up the heart and soul to experience the unity/harmony between self and God.

– No. 10 was added. Prasad - to keep the state of pleasure and a peaceful mind by becoming one with the teachings of life.

You will find great joy when you understand and practise all these teachings.

Part 3:
Releasing your body with HOGUSHI Massage

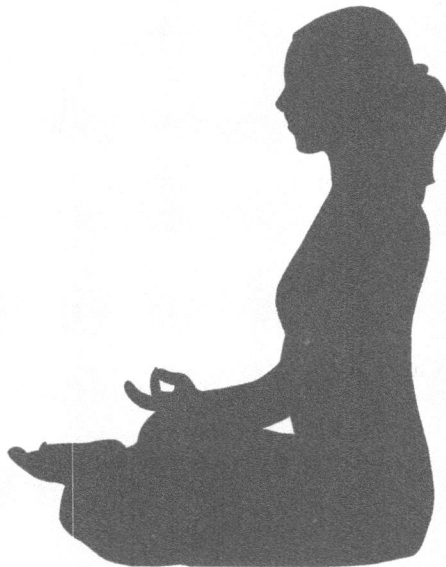

Benefits of HOGUSHI Massage before sports activities and yoga

It is important to do adequate HOGUSHI Massage before yoga and sports.

As people are normally eager to play sport or do yoga they tend to neglect warming up.

Without proper warming up, the risk of injury increases. You can apply HOGUSHI Massage as a warming up method.

It takes about 20 minutes to release the whole body including the arms, legs and lower back. Even if you are spending some time doing HOGUSHI Massage with stretching (yoga poses), it will only take around 30 to 40 minutes.

In order to play and improve skills in sport, HOGUSHI Massage has a key role.

As well as releasing the muscles prior to stretching and other warm ups, it also allows higher quality training, which assists in improving skills rapidly.

Of course the feeling of wanting more time for actual sport training to improve skills is understandable, but it is of little use if injuries occur that could be prevented.

There are many sport players who have improved their skills but had to give up their chosen sport due to injuries that originated from an inflexible body. What a waste of talent! You can avoid unnecessary injuries by gaining flexibility through daily HOGUSHI Massage (20 minutes) or combined with stretching (30 to 40 minutes). I would like to emphasise that trainers and players give it due consideration and try to use HOGUSHI Massage in their training schedule.

Benefits of HOGUSHI Massage in rehabilitation, preventing injuries and reducing pain

There are many people who need rehabilitation due to different forms of paralysis and difficulty in movement caused by illness, accidents and age. For those with rigid muscles it is an ordeal to be forced to move. With such an approach, it is difficult for them to continue rehabilitation, regardless of how much encouragement is received from doctors, physiotherapists and family members.

It is much more effective and less painful to release the stiff areas first, then gain muscle strength before actual rehabilitation.

HOGUSHI Massage is helpful in that it can create an injury and pain free body through flexibility, not only for sports, but also for simple activities such as walking. HOGUSHI Massage is also effective in its ability to avoid various occupational diseases.

Some people suffer from tenosynovitis or wrist pain from using their bodies unevenly due to the nature of their work, such as office workers using a computer and pianists.

Also, those who do handicrafts such as ceramic arts and leather crafts may suffer from ache in their shoulders and lower back.

By getting into the habit of doing HOGUSHI Massage on the areas frequently over used, before work, severe pain can be avoided. Applying HOGUSHI at the end of the day's work can also remove physical fatigue. In doing so, you are able to create a good cycle of maintenance that requires less time for releasing the muscles the following day. A huge difference can be noticed by even lightly releasing the shoulders and elbows, rather than the whole body.

It is not productive to work with pain. By reducing pain and physical fatigue, work speed is effectively enhanced. Applying HOGUSHI Massage for five to ten minutes before and after work reduces occupational posture pains and certainly makes you feel better.

DISCLAIMER

You should consult your doctor or other health adviser before doing any of the poses or exercises in this book if you have a medical condition or injury. Always disclose any medical condition or injury to your yoga teacher. Mild soreness may be experienced after yoga or other exercise; if it persists for more than 2-3 days, consult your health adviser. The author and publisher have taken care in preparing this book but accept no liability for injury or loss resulting from following its contents.

Typical body movements and the recommended HOGUSHI Massage for different sports

Baseball

Instantaneous reactions are required in baseball. Different team members such as pitchers, catchers and fielders use their bodies in different ways. There are extra impacts on the bodies of pitchers and catchers, so they should spend a little longer on HOGUSHI Massage and do poses such as Twist and Open Legged Forward Bend.

Due to the use of a dominant hand to throw balls, they should also do shadow throwing without a ball, on the opposite arm for 10 to 20 times to correct body alignment.

As the batting motion can also be a cause of distortion, then shadow batting for 10 to 20 times using the non-dominant arm would be recommended too. It is the same concept as counter balance in yoga.

Soccer

Soccer is like a combative sport, as it requires running all over the field to kick the ball and use of the upper body, including the head. It is essential to do HOGUSHI Massage and stretching for the whole body and exercises to strengthen the muscles in the legs and lower back before matches.

In soccer, players need to do HOGUSHI Massage particularly on the hips. Pigeon pose and its counter balance, the Splits, and rotating the ankles are highly recommended before matches. Also after a game apply shadow kicking without a ball using the non-dominant leg 10 to 20 times for counter balance.

It is indispensable to apply HOGUSHI Massage and stretching to maintain the body after matches. By not bothering to maintain the body after matches and training due to fatigue, there may be an escalation of conditions in the knees and lower back.

Applying HOGUSHI Massage is a "Must Do" after matches and training.

Tennis

Tennis is a sport that moves quickly over the whole court while gripping and swinging a racquet. It is highly recommended before matches to do exercises to strengthen the muscles in the arms and legs, perform rotations for the shoulders, arms, lower back and ankles, plus HOGUSHI Massage and stretching for the hips (Bow, Hook and Twist poses).

After matches, ensure you do HOGUSHI Massage and stretching on the legs and the arms.

Apply shadow swings using the non-dominant arm for 10 to 20 times. This helps to prevent tennis elbow and other avoidable injuries.

Volleyball

Volleyball is actually harder than it looks. It also requires HOGUSHI Massage on the hips, the arms and the shoulders, stretching (Fish and Bow poses) and some exercises to strengthen muscles in the lower back and arms.

Spikers should do shadow spiking using the non-dominant arm, without a ball and the same with jumping on the less used leg. Also, do some shadow serving using the non-dominant arm.

Golf

Golf seems a quiet sport, but it requires swinging a long club using the whole body. It impacts on the ankles, hip joints and around the eighth thoracic vertebra.

It is very important to do HOGUSHI Massage and stretching (Twist pose, Forward Bend, Cobra and Camel) and also some exercises to strengthen the muscles in the legs and lower back before games or competition.

Also, perform shadow swings, without a ball, using the non-dominant arm for 10 to 20 times as well as HOGUSHI Massage and stretching after a game.

Jogging/Walking

It is important to do HOGUSHI Massage on the hips, rotation of the ankles and stretching the legs and the lower back (Camel pose, Open Legged Forward Bend, Splits). Also ensure to stretch the Achilles' tendons well, before and after the main exercise.

HOGUSHI Massage for various occupations

Seated work such as deskwork and handicrafts

People who do computer work all day or handicrafts for a long time impact the neck, shoulders and lower back. By applying HOGUSHI Massage on the shoulders and shoulder blades while sitting on the edge of a chair, while tucking the pelvis in and activating the abdominal region, pain and discomfort are reduced and work can continue longer.

Additionally, as the fingers tend to be facing downwards all the time, it is effective to release the shoulders, rotate the arms and bend the fingers backwards (see Figure 5).

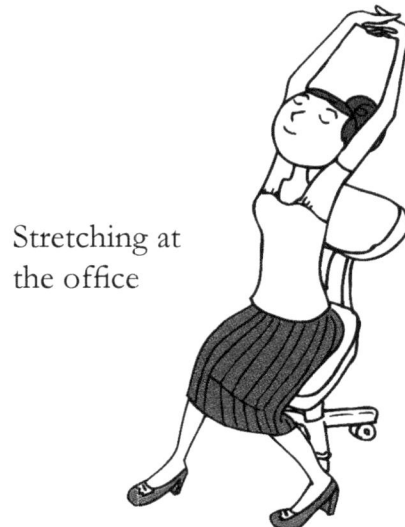

Stretching at the office

Figure 5

Standing work

People involved in standing work for long periods of time such as salespersons, chefs and nurses have tight pelvic areas and stressed knees. It is necessary to release not only the legs, but also the hips.

Farming

Some farmers gradually become stooped due to forward bending postures required by their type of work over a long period of time. It is also common for damage to their knees and lower back.

Back bend pose and releasing the hips helps to reduce the pain in the knees and lower back.

Physical Work

People involved in physical work such as construction sites, in freight and the moving industries are better to apply HOGUSHI Massage and stretching to the whole body. Ensure the shoulder blades, the hips and legs are worked thoroughly.

On the following pages the way to perform HOGUSHI Massage and Counter Balances are clearly explained with photos and illustrations.

Please practise them!

It is recommended HOGUSHI Massage and stretching positions are practised before doing the following major sports and activities:

Tennis
Bow, Plough, Hook, Twist, Standing Back Bend

Baseball
Twist, Open Legged Forward Bend, Cobra, Pigeon, Standing Back Bend

Soccer
Pigeon, Butterfly Forward Bend, Splits, Head Stand, Lotus

Volleyball
Fish, Bow, Splits, Lotus

Golf
Twist, Forward Bend, Cobra, Camel, Pigeon

Jogging / Walking
Camel, Splits, Pigeon, Shoulder Stand, Head Stand

Desk Work
Camel, Bow, Cat, Locust, Bridge

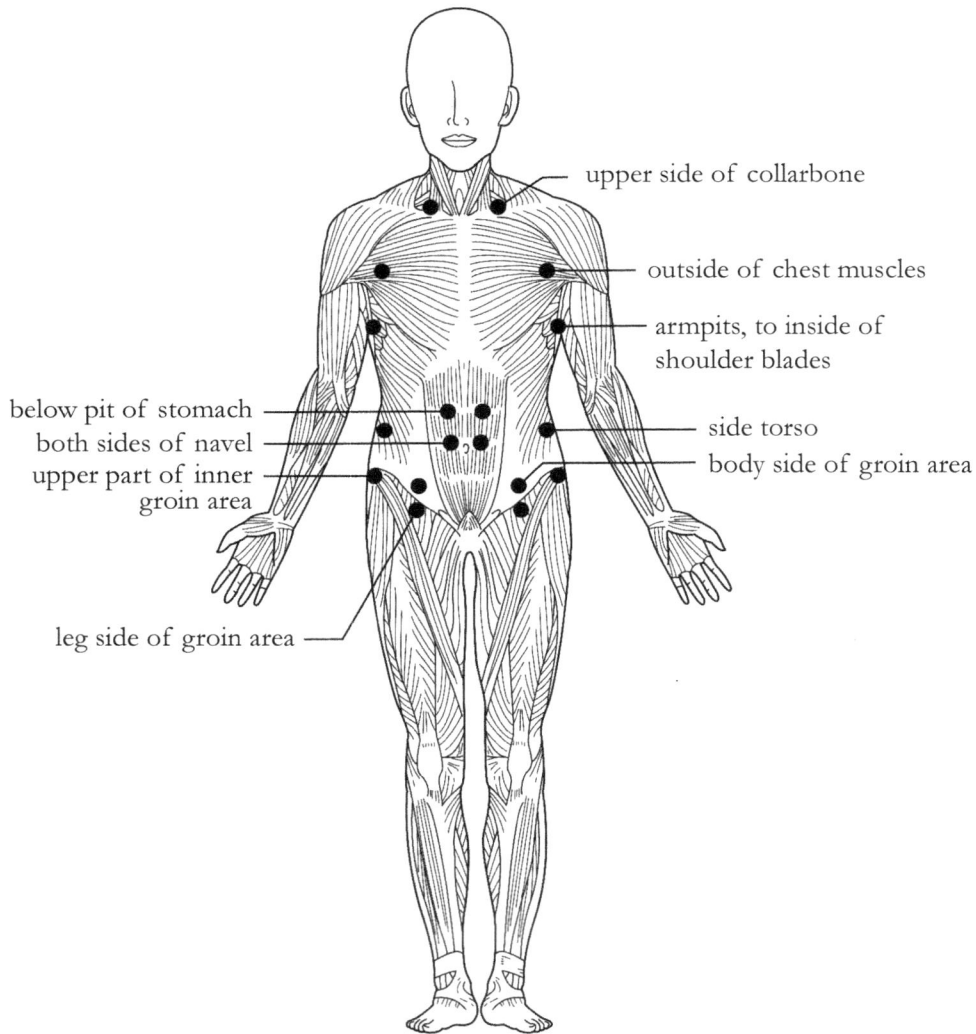

FRONT

upper side of collarbone

outside of chest muscles

armpits, to inside of
shoulder blades

below pit of stomach
both sides of navel
upper part of inner
    groin area

side torso

body side of groin area

leg side of groin area

Part
3
Releasing your body with HOGUSHI Massage

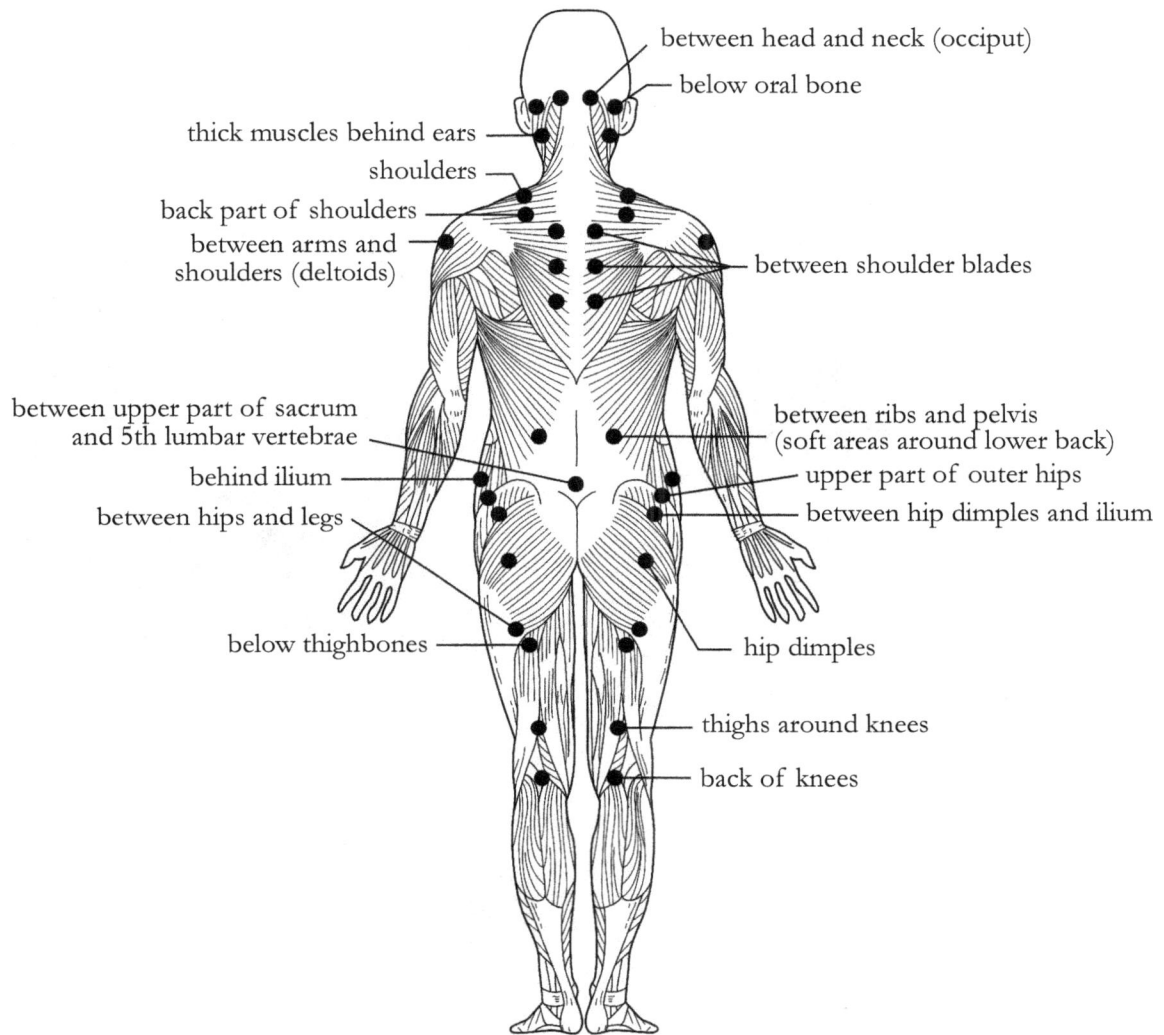

BACK

between head and neck (occiput)

below oral bone

thick muscles behind ears

shoulders

back part of shoulders

between arms and
shoulders (deltoids)

between shoulder blades

between upper part of sacrum
and 5th lumbar vertebrae

between ribs and pelvis
(soft areas around lower back)

behind ilium

upper part of outer hips

between hips and legs

between hip dimples and ilium

below thighbones

hip dimples

thighs around knees

back of knees

Hips HOGUSHI Massage
(Aim for approximately 20 to 30 repetitions)

1. On the borderline between hips and legs

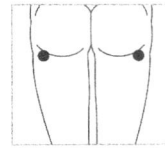

❶ In a seated position with the legs outstretched, place the soles of the feet together and lean the body forwards to grasp feet.

❷ Rock from side-to-side using the body weight on the area, between hips and legs.

❸ Rock the area backward and forward using body weight.

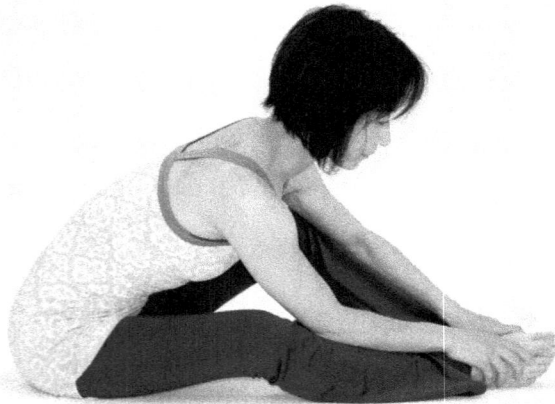

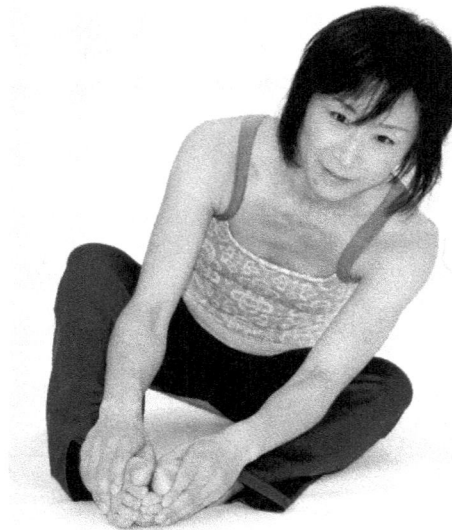

2. Hip dimples

❶ Place hands behind the body to position the hip dimples on the ground and rock the area side-to-side and back to front.

❷ Do the same on the other side.

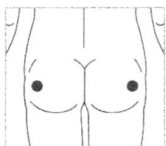

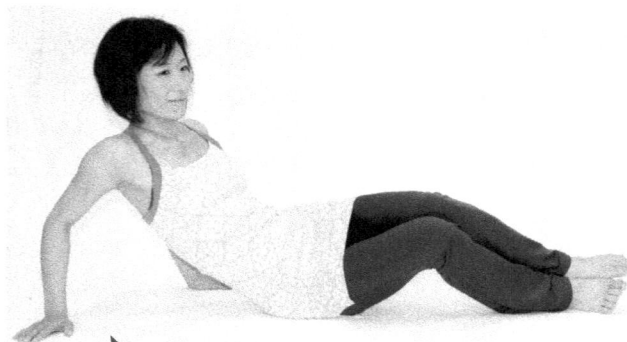

hands support the position

3. Between hip dimple and ilium

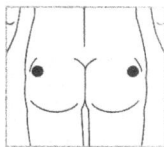

❶ Place the right hand diagonally behind the body and left hand to the front of hips to support the body.

❷ Adjust the position of left knee (top knee) to support the body.

❸ Adjust the position of right knee (bottom knee) to allow the targeted area to touch the ground.

❹ Rock the area side-to-side and back and front.

❺ Do the other side.

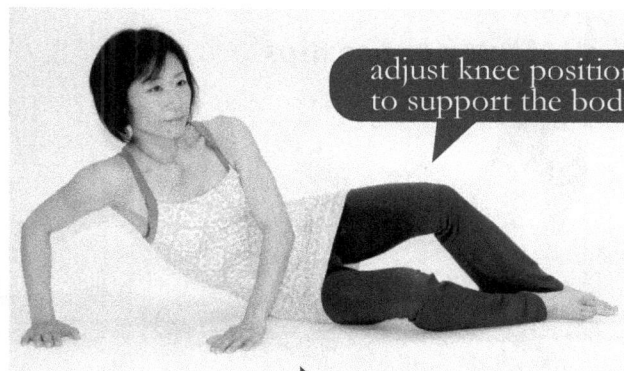

adjust knee position to support the body

slightly bend elbow

4. Upper outer hips

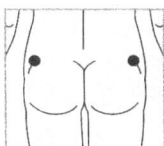

❶ From the position made in No. 3, place the right elbow on the ground to support upper body.

❷ Place the upper outer hip (above No. 3) on the ground and rock the area side to side and back to front. It would be easier to rock back to front with the lower leg stretched and to rock side-to-side with slight tensing of the inner knee in the upright leg.

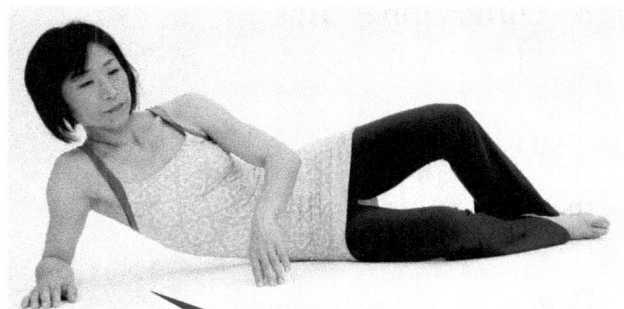

❸ Do the other side.

bend elbow to support the body

5. Behind ilium

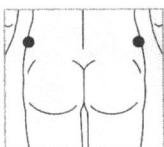

❶ From the position of No. 4, place the right elbow further away from body and lean back.

❷ Place the upper outer hip and back of the pelvis on the ground and rock the area side-to-side and back to front.

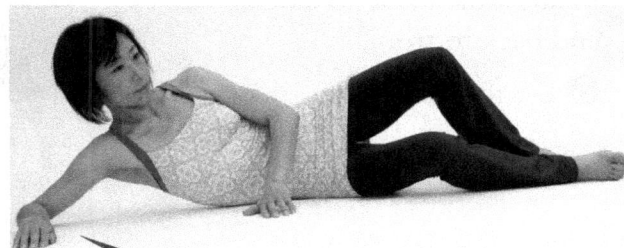

❸ Do the other side.

place elbow further away from body

Point: While releasing the area from the bottom of hips to the upper hips through No. 2 to No. 5, be aware of targeted areas.

Note: Please adjust the number of repetitions in terms of pain and stiffness.

6. Outer upper hips

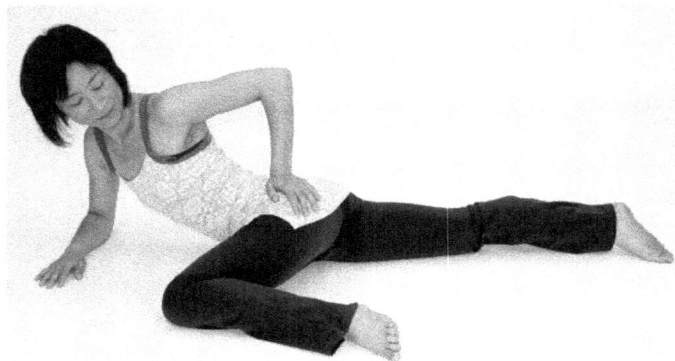

❶ Lie on the stomach and place right elbow on the ground to support the upper body.

❷ Pull the left knee to the side of the body and massage the outer upper hip with left hand.

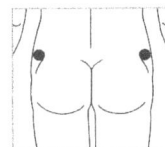

❸ Do the other side.

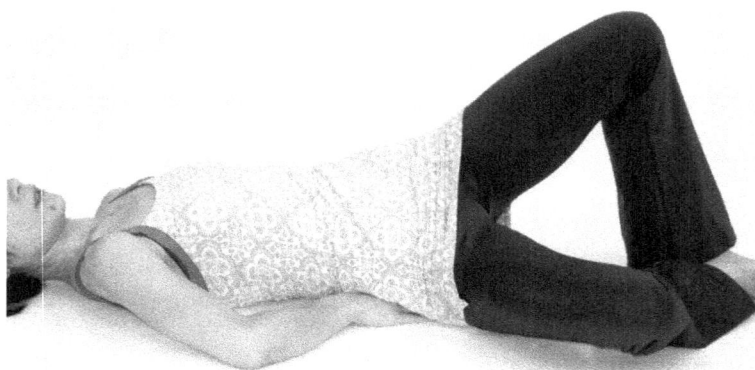

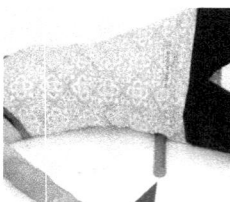

7. Outer upper hips

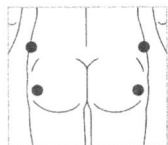

the spots to place hands

❶ Place feet together and lift left hip up.

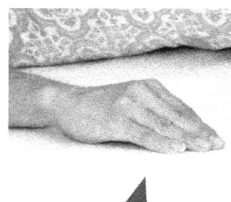

❷ Place mountain shaped knuckle to touch the muscle under right thigh bone and rock the area side-to-side and back to front.

❸ Do the other side.

wooden rod

mountain shaped knuckle

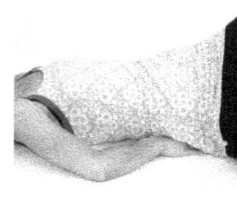

Point:
★ As a variation, place mountain shaped knuckle under the leg side of groin bone.
★ Use a wooden rod under thigh bone as a substitute for knuckle.

Legs HOGUSHI Massage
(Aim for 20 times each)

1. Under the thighbones & on the thigh muscles in buttock crease to the back of knee

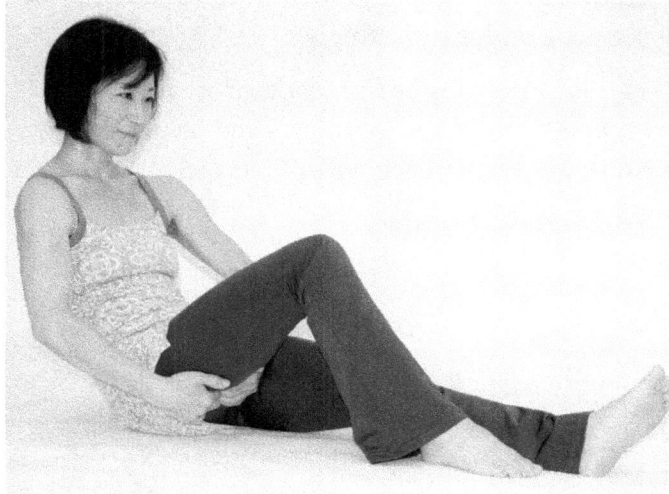

❶ Lift right knee up, place 8 fingers (without thumbs) between hip and leg tendons and massage the area and muscles side-to-side.

❷ Place 6 fingers (without thumbs and little fingers) on the back of thigh and massage the area from the buttock crease to the back of knee.

❸ Do the other side.

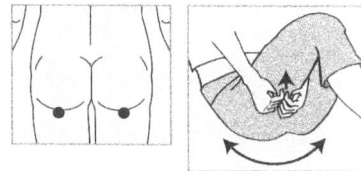

2. Back of the knees

❶ Place thumbs on the back of right knee and slide them from upper part to lower part of the area along the muscle.

❷ Do the other side.

NOTE: Do not apply this on the calves.

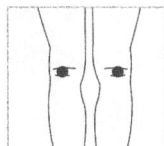

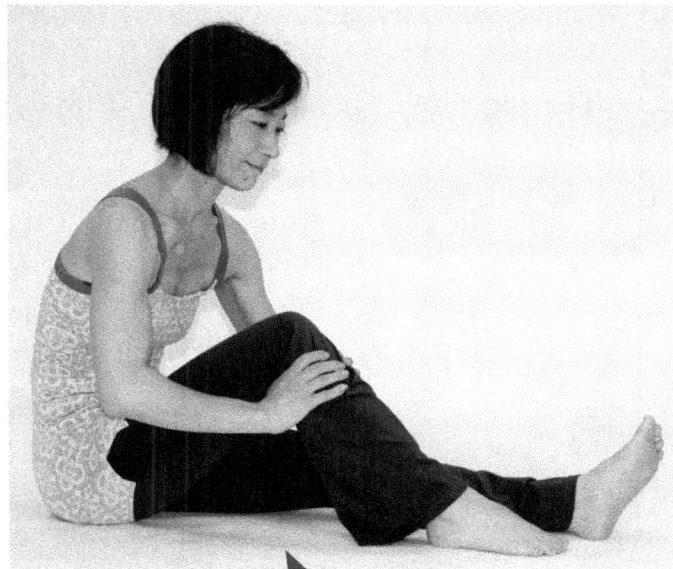

sliding fingers from upper part to lower part

Groin Area HOGUSHI Massage

(Aim for 10 times each)

1. Groin Area

❶ Straighten right leg, bend left leg and slide the foot under right thigh.

❷ Place thumbs at right side of groin area (between body and right leg) and apply finger pressure towards the anus.

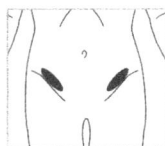

❸ Do the other side.

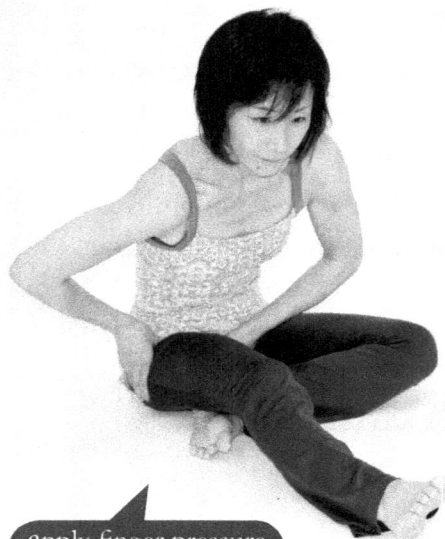

apply finger pressure towards the anus (not towards legs)

Point: By placing the bent leg under the straightened leg, it makes it easier to apply finger pressure as the area is more relaxed.

Note: Ensure to apply finger pressure towards the anus to be effective or it will not work.

2. The leg side of groin areas I

slightly bend the knees outward when massaging

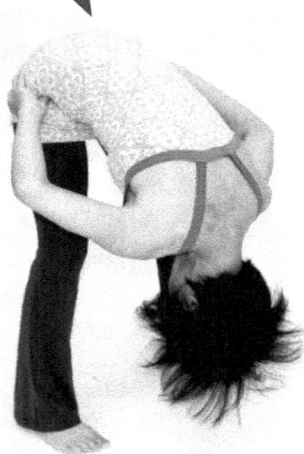

Place thumbs below ilium and find the spot, which stiffens when raising the body and softens when bending the body. Bend the knees slightly and bend the body forward to apply finger pressure on the soft spots.

3. Leg side of groin areas II

❶ Be in the same posture as 1-1.

❷ Relax the thick tendon below ilium (the area that stands out when the leg is straightened and ankle raised). Apply finger pressure and also shake the area.

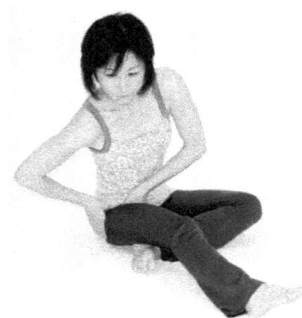

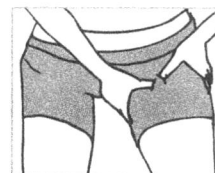

❸ Do the other side.

Part 3 Releasing your body with HOGUSHI Massage

Side of the Torso HOGUSHI Massage
(Aim for 10 times each side)

1.

Place thumbs between ilium and ribs and apply finger pressure.

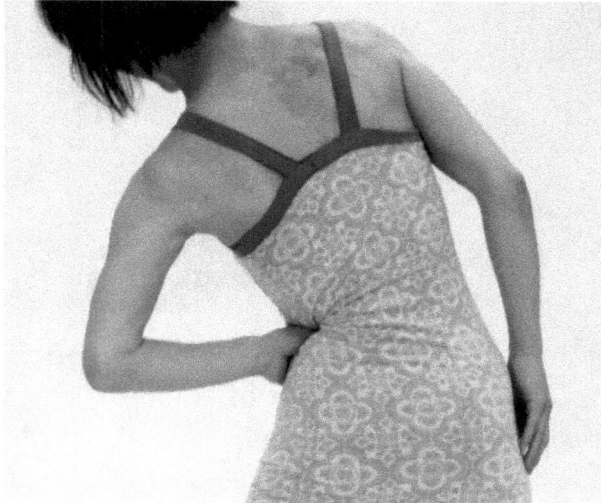

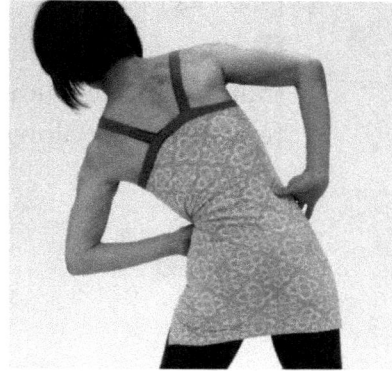

Point:
By releasing the area between the ilium and ribs, it will be easier to stretch the side of the body.

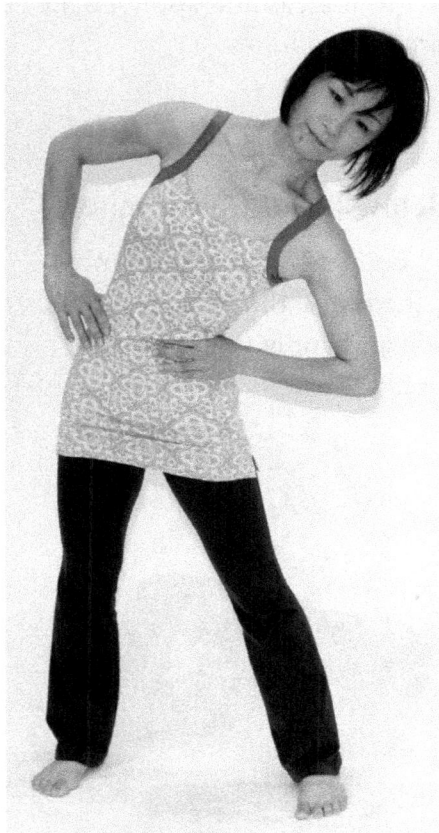

2.

For people with a stiff body, apply finger pressure to the contracted side in a gentle side bend.

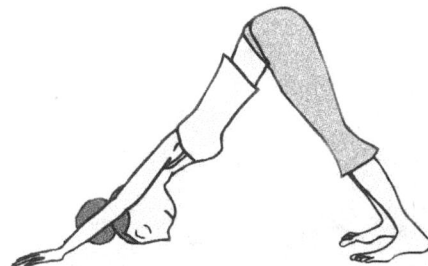

Easing the side and the groin areas helps with Down Facing Dog pose.

Abdomen HOGUSHI Massage

(Aim for 10 times each)

1. Body side of the groin areas

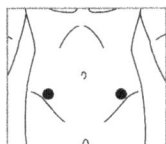

❶ Bend the knees slightly and place feet together.

❷ Place 8 fingers (excluding thumbs) inside ilium and apply finger pressure along the pelvis.

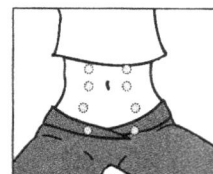

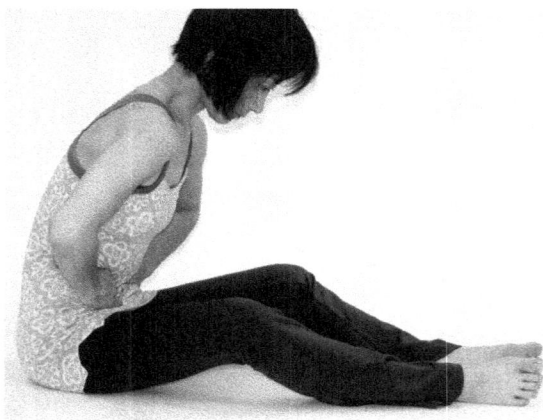

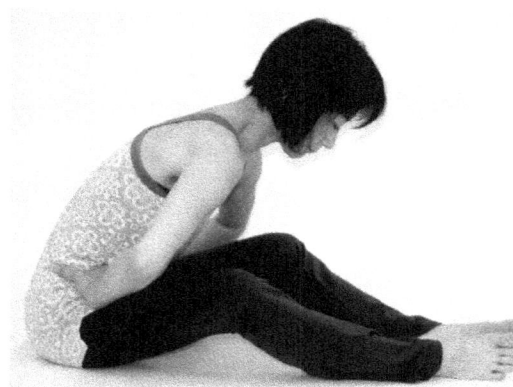

2. Upper part of inner groin area

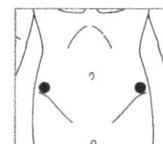

In the same position, place 8 fingers on the upper body side of groin areas and apply finger pressure along ilium.

3. Sides of the navel

Place 8 fingers (excluding thumbs) on either side of the navel and apply finger pressure.

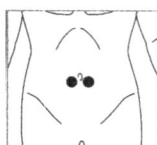

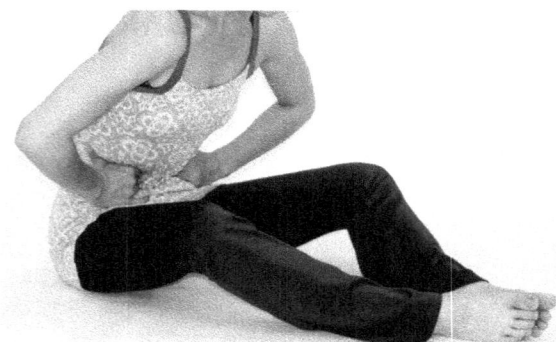

4. Below pit of the stomach

Place 8 fingers (excluding thumbs) below the pit of the stomach and apply finger pressure.

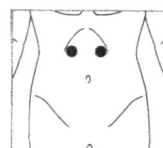

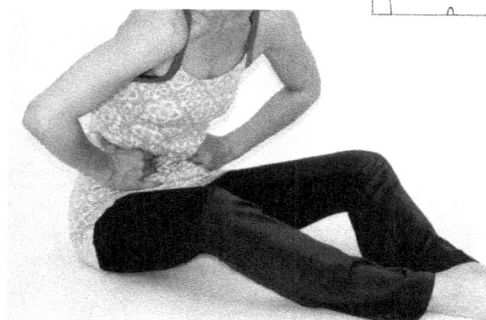

Point: Relax the whole torso throughout the massage, 1 to 4.

Part 3 Releasing your body with HOGUSHI Massage

Lower Back HOGUSHI Massage
(Aim for 10 times each)

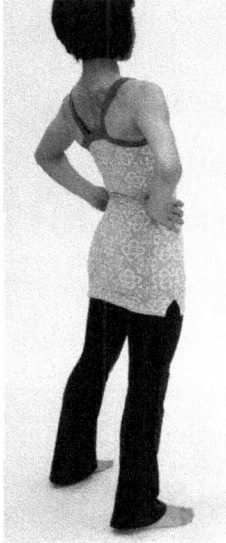

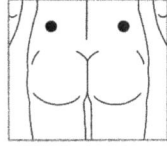

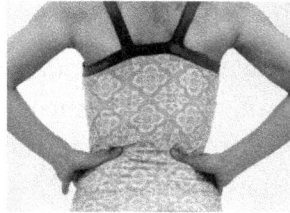

1. Between the ribs and the pelvis

❶ In a standing position, bend the knees slightly and tuck the pelvis under to push the belly out.

❷ Place the hands on the hips with thumbs on the soft muscle between the ribs and the pelvis and apply finger pressure.

Point: The thumbs should sink into the waist cavity naturally in the position made in 1.1.

2. Between upper part of sacrum and the 5th lumber vertebrae – I

In the same position made in 1-1, place thumbs between the upper part of sacrum and the 5th lumber vertebrae and apply finger pressure.

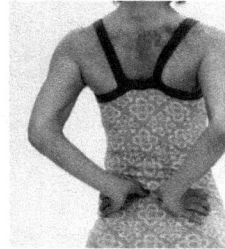

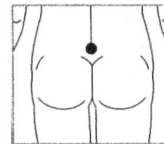

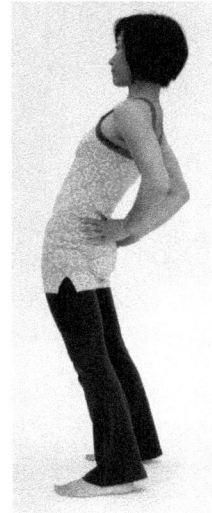

3. Between upper part of sacrum & 5th lumber vertebrae–II

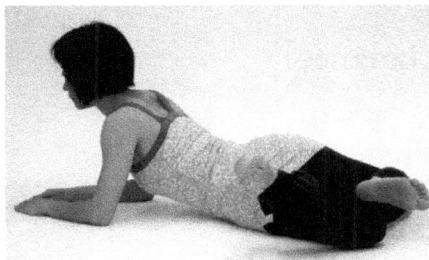

❶ Lie on the stomach, place elbows on the ground in line with shoulders to support the upper body and bend knees to point the feet to the sky.

❷ Keep the knees together and rhythmically swing feet side to side.

Point: With the upper body raised while swinging the feet, the back muscles tend to be released.

4. Between upper part of sacrum and the 5th lumber vertebrae – III

❶ Lie on the stomach and place the hands under the chin. Tuck toes under.

❷ Press the knees to the ground to raise the hips and hold this posture for several seconds.

❸ Relax hips back on the ground.

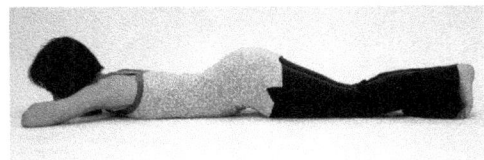

Shoulder Blades HOGUSHI Massage

(Aim for 10 times each)

1. Between shoulder blades 1

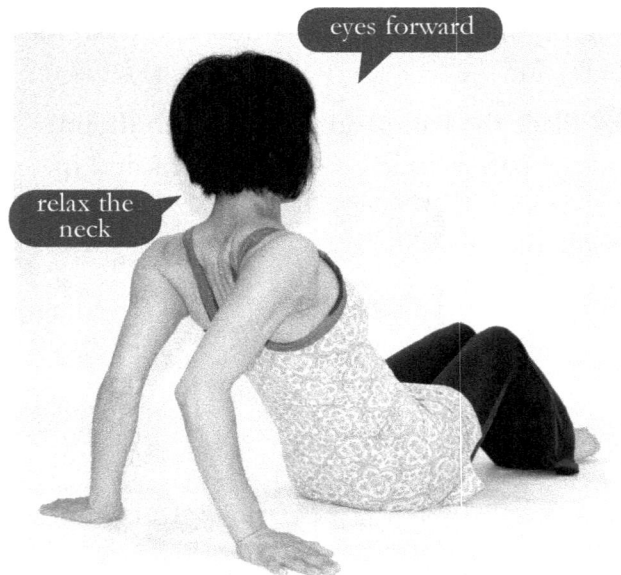

eyes forward

relax the neck

fingers facing backward, or facing out to the sides if necessary

❶ From a seated position, raise the knees and place the palms behind the body. Squeeze the shoulder blades toward each other while opening the chest

❷ Repeat squeezing and separating them like a fluttering butterfly.

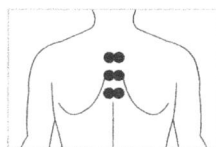

Point: For beginners, if moving both shoulder blades is difficult, do one side at a time. When you are comfortable with the movement, do both together, similar to a fluttering butterfly.

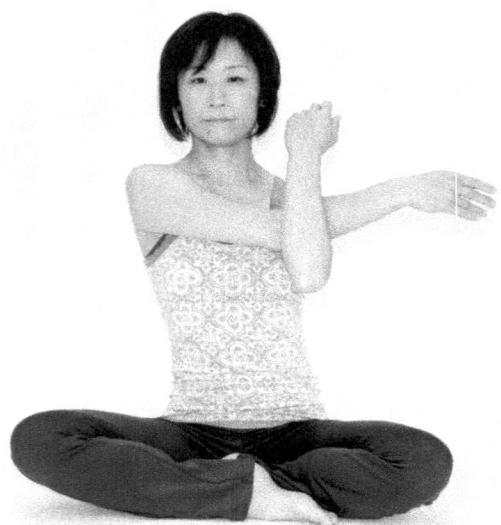

2. Counter balance

❶ As a counter balance to 1, cross one arm over the front of the body to widen the shoulder blade.

❷ Do the other side.

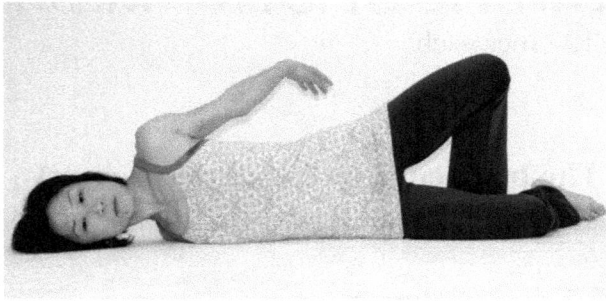

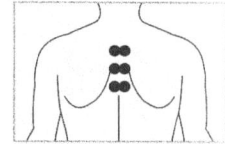

3. Between shoulder blades 2

❶ Lie on one side and place the bottom shoulder to the ground stretching it backwards.

❷ Gently rock the area side-to-side and back to front.

❸ Do the other side.

> **Point:** For people having difficulty with this posture, an alternative is to place the bottom arm under the head as a pillow and rock the area.

4. Counter balance 1

❶ Lie on one side and place the bottom arm stretched out from the front of the body.

❷ Roll the body on to the stomach over the outstretched arm. This will stretch the other side of the arm muscles and widen the shoulder blades.

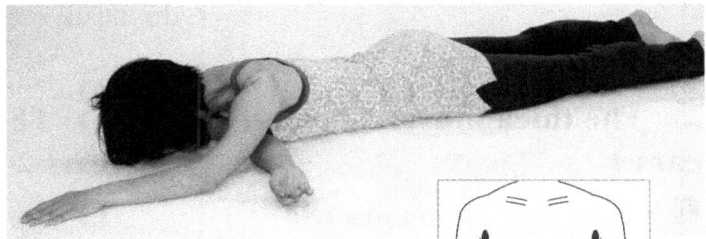

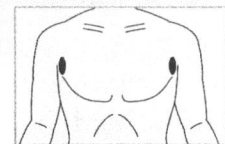

outside of chest muscles

5. Counter balance 2

❶ From the position made in 3, bend the top knee and place the foot on the ground (behind the bottom leg).

❷ Stretch the bottom arm behind the torso, palm facing up. Place the upper arm parallel to the lower arm, palm facing down.

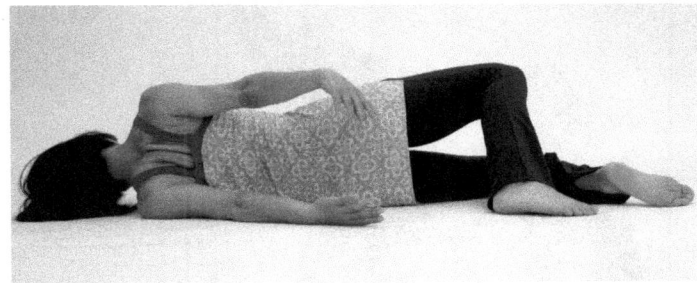

❸ Open the chest aiming to have the face close to the ground.

❹ Rock the chest back and forth, aiming to bring the chest to the ground. Use body weight to help the movement.

❺ Repeat on the other side.

Neck & back of the Head HOGUSHI Massage

(Aim for 10 times each)

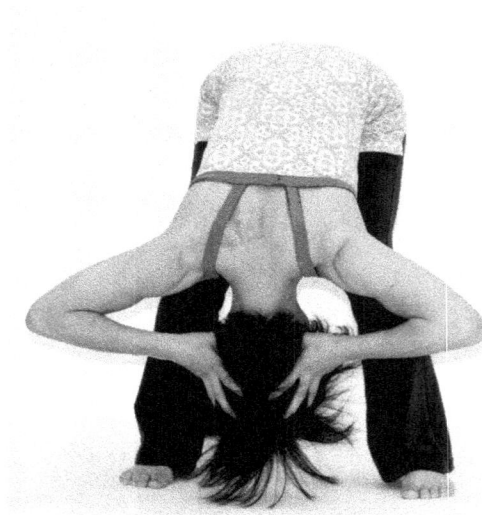

1. The back edge of the skull (occiput) & Between the neck and the head

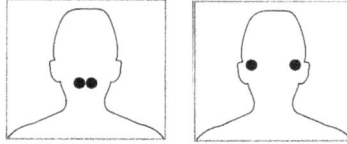

❶ In a standing position with feet waist width apart, bend forward.

❷ Hold the head with hands and massage the target areas, the back edge of the skull and between the neck and the head.

> **Point:** In a Forward Bend position, the neck and surrounding areas will be released easily.

2. The thick muscles behind the ears 1

❶ Stay in the position made in No 1, massage the thick muscles behind the ears.

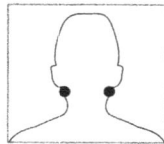

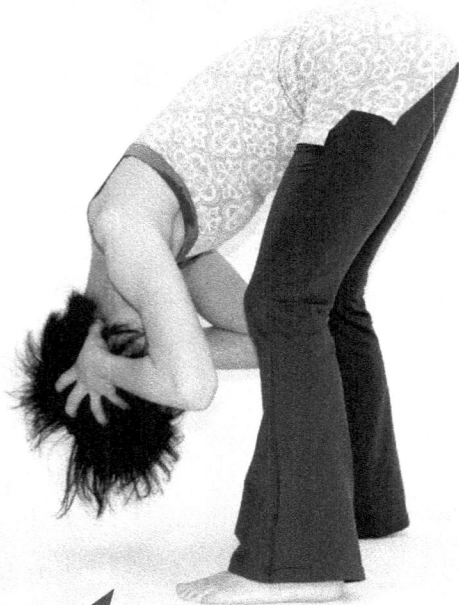

> for people having difficulty keeping this position, it is alright to bend the knees

3. The thick muscles behind the ears 2

❶ Cup left palm under the chin and push the chin to the side to relax the back of the neck.

❷ Use the right hand to assist stretching the neck and to massage the back of the neck.

❸ Repeat on the other side.

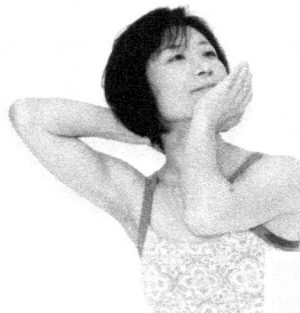

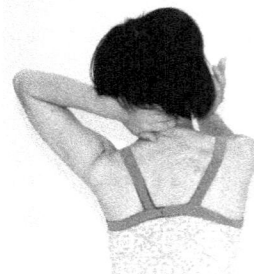

Shoulders & Arms HOGUSHI Massage

(Aim for 10 times each. Repeat if stiffness remains.)

1. Along the upper side of collarbone

❶ Place the right elbow on a platform, such as a chair, with the level of slightly higher than the shoulder height to support the arm.

❷ With the left hand, massage along the upper side of the collarbone area using 3 fingers (except thumb and little finger), with the feeling of reaching under the collarbone.

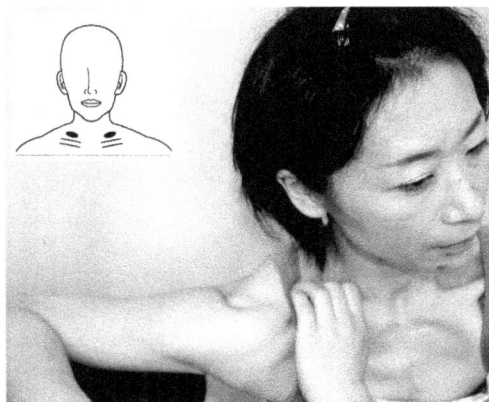

2. Between the shoulders and the arms

Place fingers in the joint area between the shoulder and arm, shaking the area back and forth.

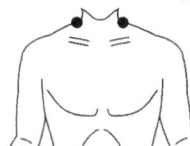 eyes forward

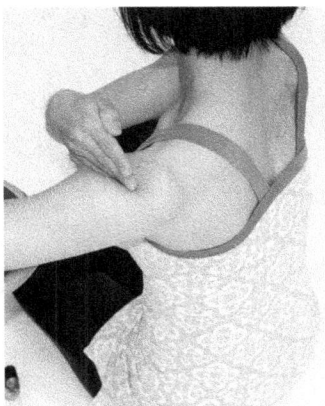

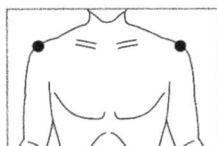

3. Shoulders

Massage the muscles between the shoulders and arms while moving the shoulder joints up and down.

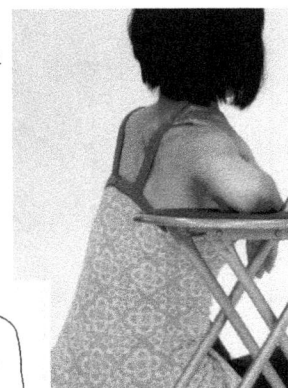

4. Between the armpit and the inner side of shoulder blade

Pinch and massage the muscles between the armpits and shoulder blades using the thumb and fingers.

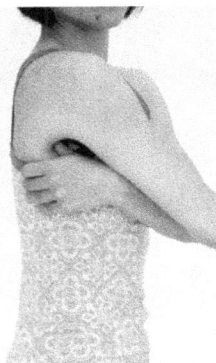

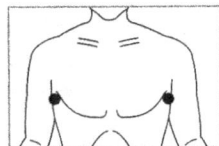

5.

Do 1 to 4 on one side and repeat on the other side.

Point:

★ It is easier to release the area while exhaling as the shoulders are more relaxed.

★ Use a drawn up knee as a platform when a chair is not available.

Lower Back Counter Balance

(Aim for 2 to 3 times)

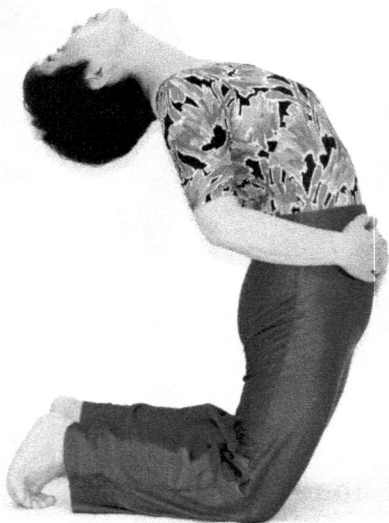

1. Camel Pose

❶ In a kneeling position with the knees waist width apart, place the palms on the lower belly.

❷ Tuck the pelvis in and lean back slightly. Open the chest and push the chin up to the sky with taking the arms over head, interlacing fingers.

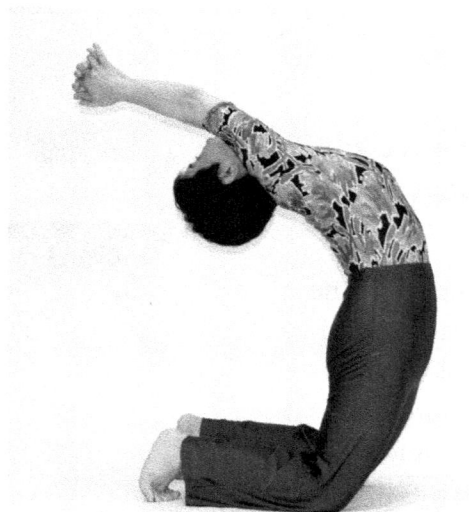

Point:
This is a counter balance for Forward Bend poses.

2. Boat Pose

❶ Lie on the back and hold the knees with interlaced fingers.

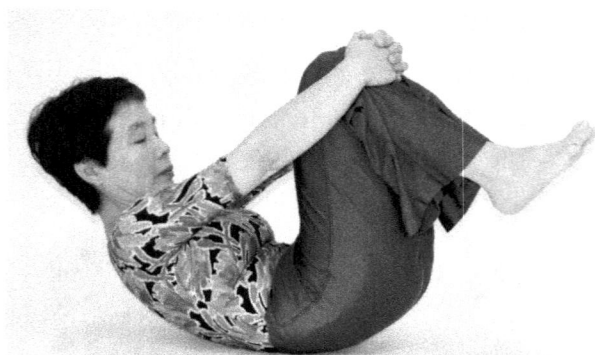

❷ Tuck the chin in

Point:
This counter balance is good after any Bend Over poses as the spine curls and the shoulder blades open.

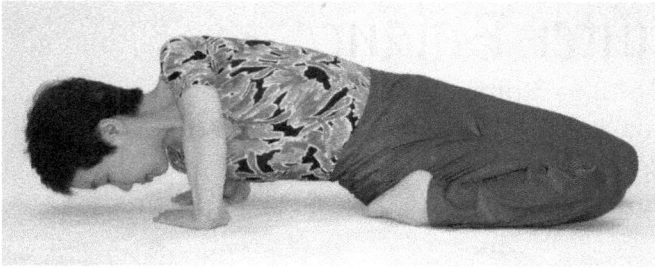

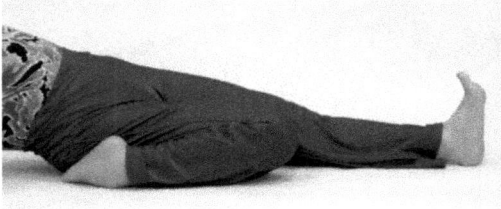

3. Twist in the Hero Pose

❶ In the Hero pose, place the heels beside the hips.

❷ Twist the upper body and lean backward with the aim of placing the palms behind the body.

Point:

★ By twisting, the muscles around the hips are released. The closer the face reaches the ground, the more the hips are released.

★ For people having difficulty in this seated position, it is alright to straighten one leg.

4. Cat Pose

❶ Come onto all fours, with the hips above the knees and the hands directly below the shoulders.

❷ Tuck the chin in, curl the spine upward to look at the belly button.

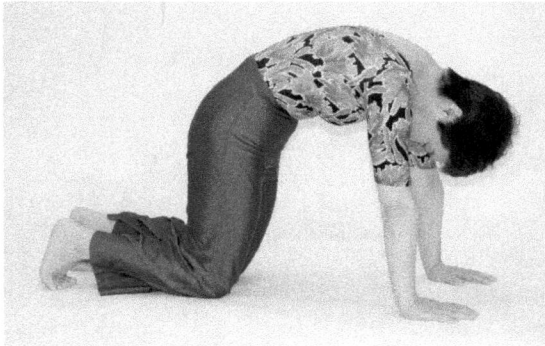

5. Standing Forward Bend

❶ Stand with the feet waist width apart.

❷ Bend forward, using body weight to create the stretch.

❸ Hold the back of the legs.

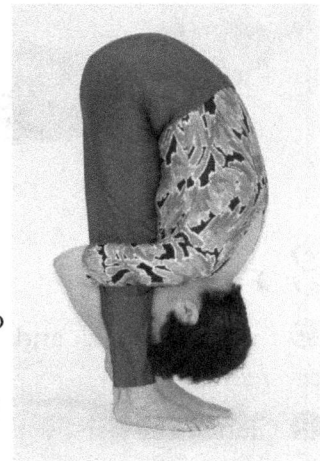

Point:

This counter balance is good after any Back Bend poses.

6. Standing Back Bend Pose

❶ Stand with the feet waist width apart, place the palms on the lower back.

❷ Bend the knees slightly and tuck the pelvis in.

❸ Raise the chest and open the chin to the sky.

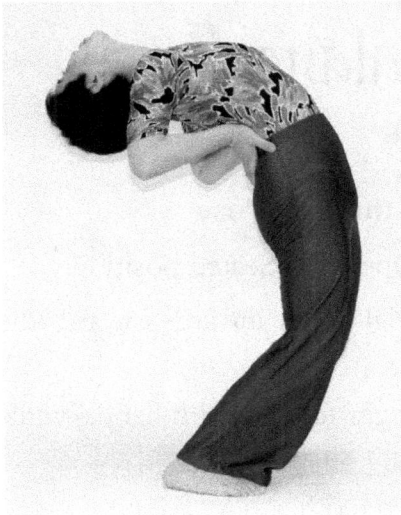

Neck Counter Balance

(Aim for 2 to 3 times)

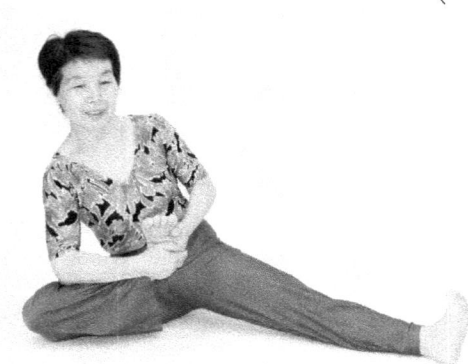

1. Fish Pose 1

❶ Lie on the back and slide the hands under the hips, dorsiflexing the feet.

❷ Raise the chest, tilt the head and open the chin to the sky.

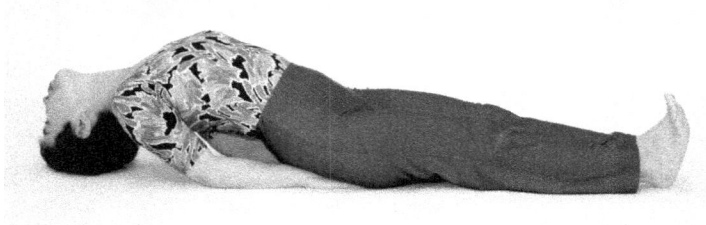

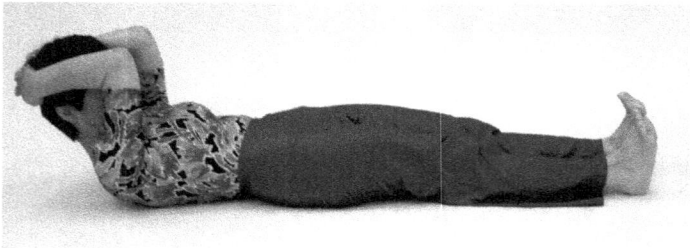

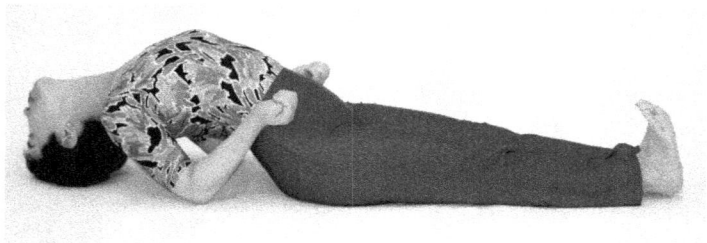

2. Neck Stretch Pose

❶ Lie on the back and dorsiflex the feet.

❷ Hold the back of the head and with grasped hands and tuck the chin in, stretch the back of the neck.

3. Fish Pose 2

❶ Lie on the back and dorsiflex the feet.

❷ Clench the fists, with thumbs on the inside and place the elbows on the ground beside ribs.

❸ Raise the chest, tilt the head and open the chin to the sky.

Knees Counter Balance

(Aim for 2 to 3 times)

1. Holding the Leg Pose

❶ Sit in an Open Leg Seated position.

❷ Bend the right knee inwards towards the groin.

❸ Hold the right foot up with hands, while placing the right knee on the ground.

❹ Repeat on the other side.

Part 3 Releasing your body with HOGUSHI Massage

Finding suitable stretches and HOGUSHI Massage for personal use

Yoga poses (asanas) work to effectively stretch the whole body. They help to improve the blood flow and by addition of HOGUSHI Massage, help to reduce pain and make the body more flexible.

On the following pages are some yoga poses with the HOGUSHI Massage to do before practicing the poses and Counter Balances recommended after. Repeat the cycles shown as a set, for at least five sets.

Refer back to the previous section on the recommended poses for different sports and types of work. Please experiment to find your own combinations so that you are able to relieve your condition with HOGUSHI Massage and stretching. Even people who play the same sport will have individual variations of distortion or stiffness in their bodies. It does not matter if you are different from the majority of people; just do your own version of HOGUSHI Massage and stretching for your individual needs.

To find the appropriate HOGUSHI Massage and stretching for yourself; listen to your body carefully, to pin point the source of the discomfort or pain.

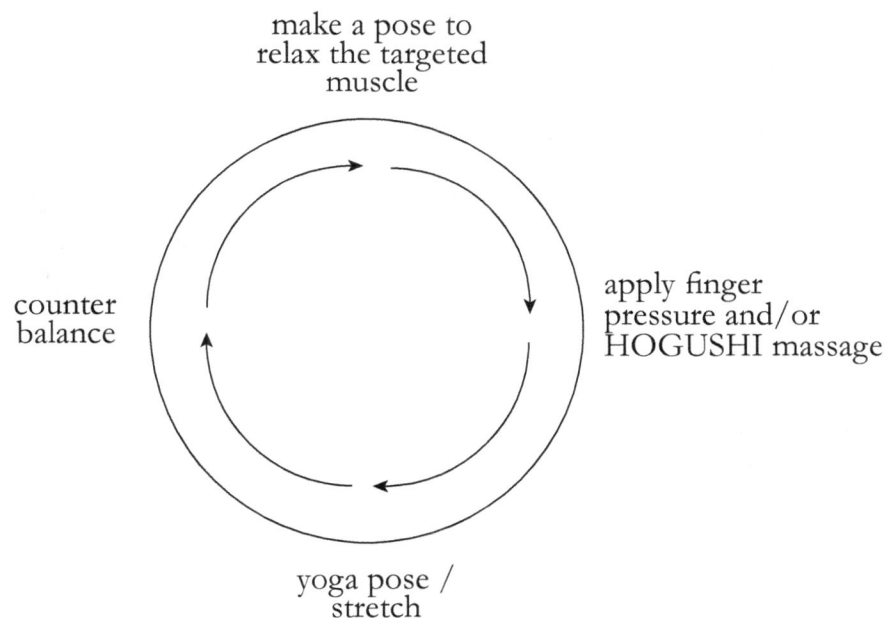

make a pose to
relax the targeted
muscle

counter
balance

apply finger
pressure and/or
HOGUSHI massage

yoga pose /
stretch

Figure 6:
Repeat this pattern as a set
for at least 5 sets.

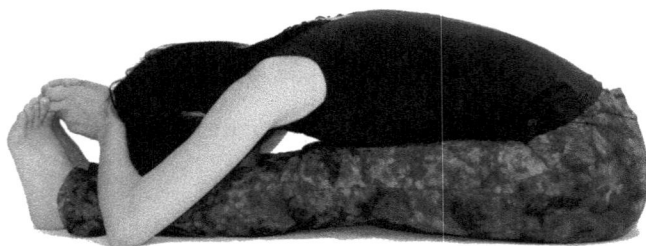

Forward Bend

Effect: Stretches the back of the legs and the lower back. Recover from fatigue.

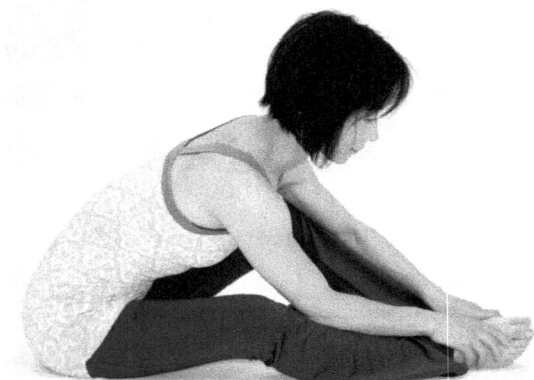

1. Hips 1 HOGUSHI Massage (p40-41)

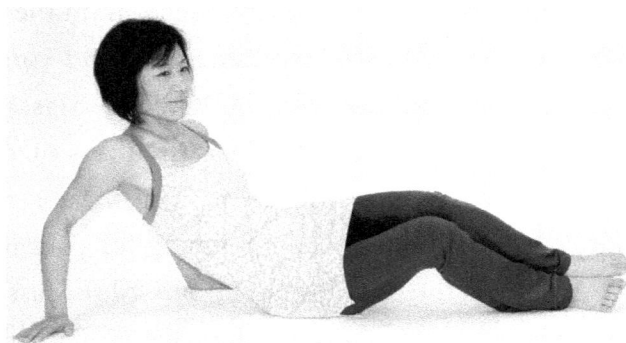

2. Hips 2 HOGUSHI Massage

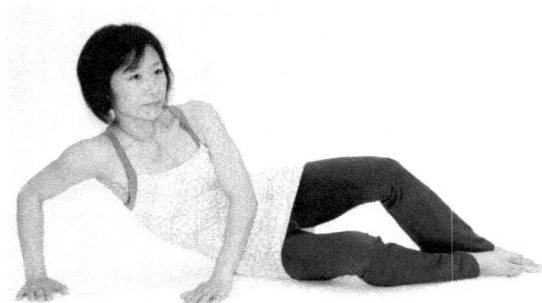

3. Hips 3 HOGUSHI Massage

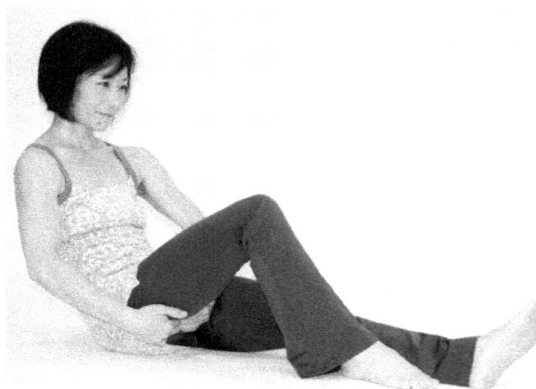

4. Legs 1 HOGUSHI Massage (p43)

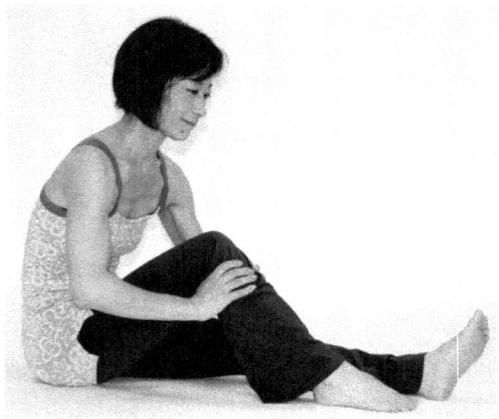

5. Legs 2 HOGUSHI Massage

Part 3 Releasing your body with HOGUSHI Massage

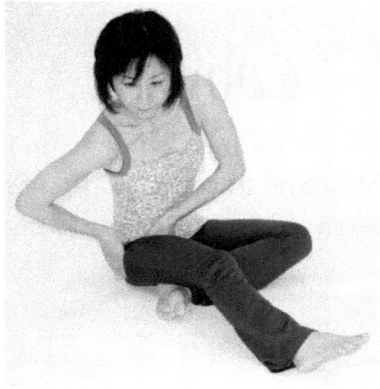

6. Groin Area 3
HOGUSHI Massage (p44)

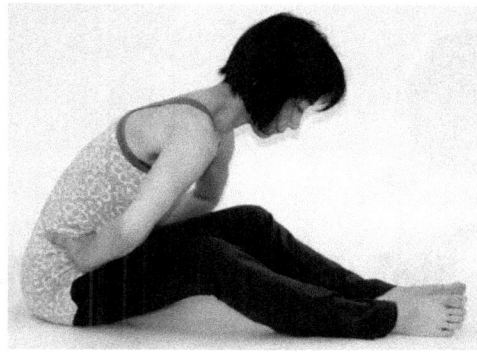

7. Abdomen 2 HOGUSHI Massage (p46)

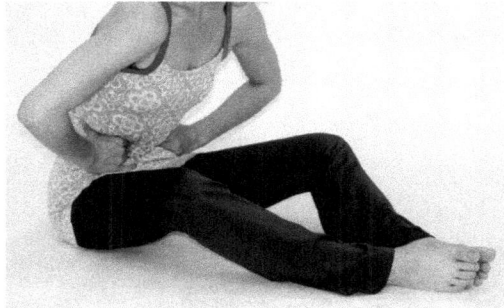

8. Abdomen 3 HOGUSHI Massage

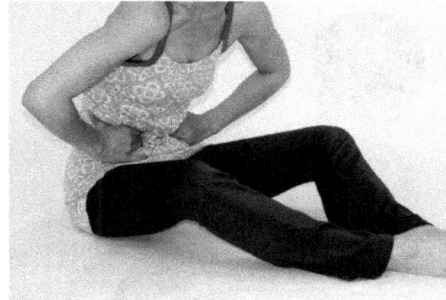

9. Abdomen 4 HOGUSHI Massage

10. Forward Bend

In a seated position, straighten the legs and bend forward, with the aim of touching the torso / chest to the thighs and the face close to the ankles.

Point

3 typical reasons make it difficult to do a Forward Bend:

1. Because the hips are stiff, the legs do not straighten.

2. Because the back of the knees are stiff, the knees do not stay on the ground.

3. Because the torso is stiff, the body does not bend forward.

It is important to apply HOGUSHI Massage on the hips, the back of the knees and the abdomen.

AFTER THE POSE

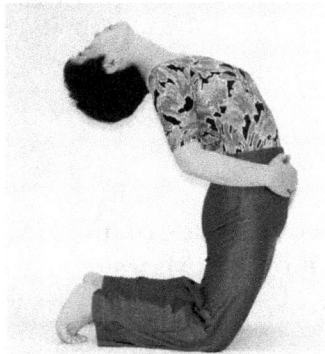

1. Lower Back 1
Counter Balance (p52)

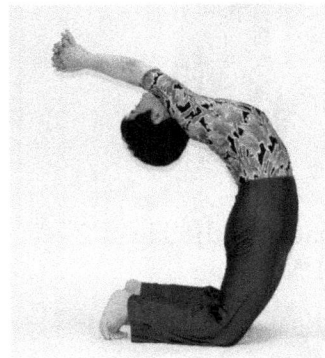

2. Lower Back 2
Counter Balance

Stretching & HOGUSHI Massage

Cobra

Effect: Remove muscle fatigue in the back, chest and lower back. Increase flexibility in the lower back and neck.

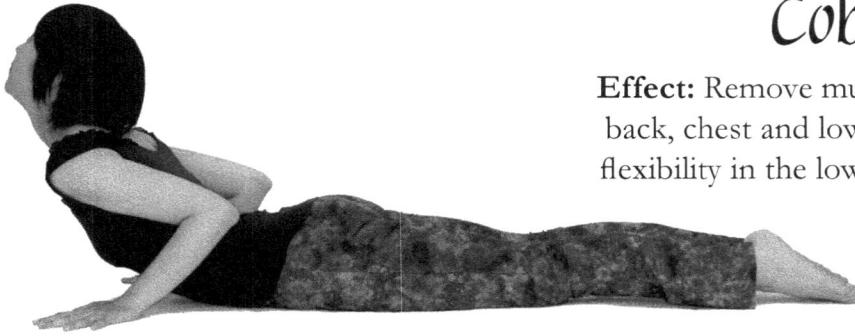

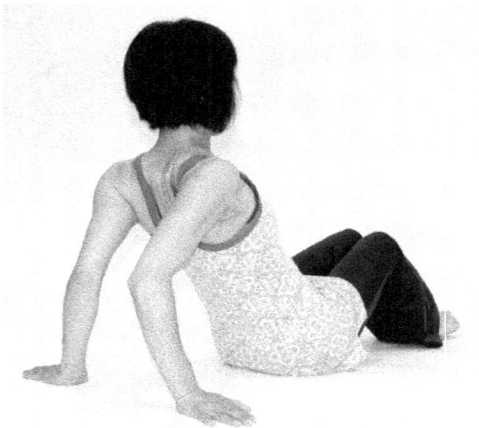

1. Shoulder Blades 1
   HOGUSHI Massage (p48)

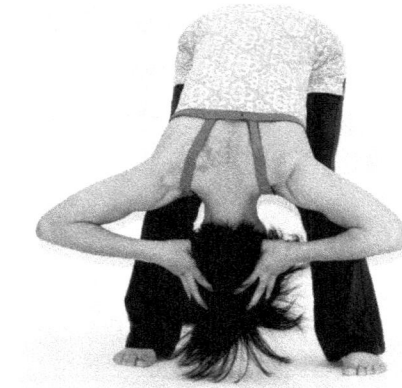

2. Neck and back of the Head 1
   HOGUSHI Massage (p50)

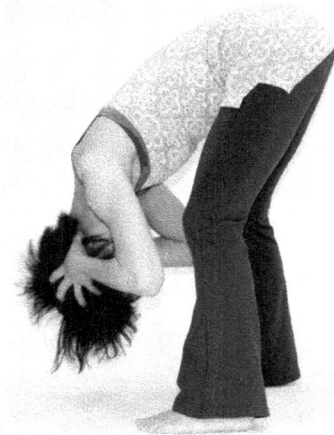

3. Neck and back of the Head 2
   HOGUSHI Massage

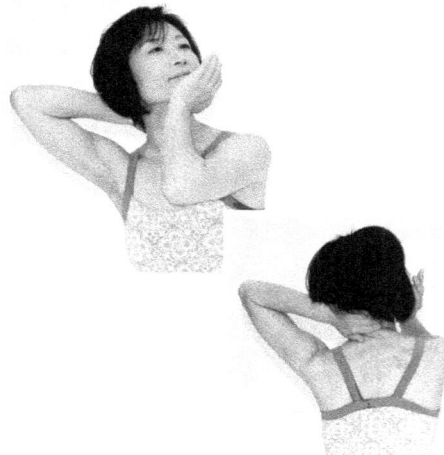

4. Neck and back of the Head 3
   HOGUSHI Massage

5.

Lower Back 1
HOGUSHI Massage
(p47)

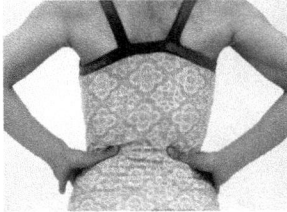

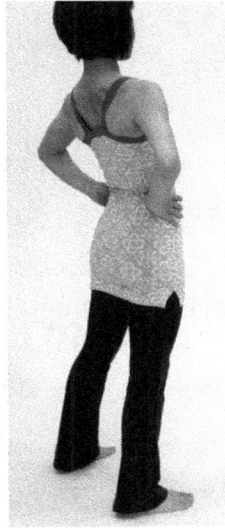

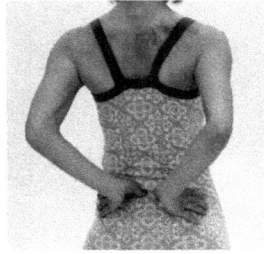

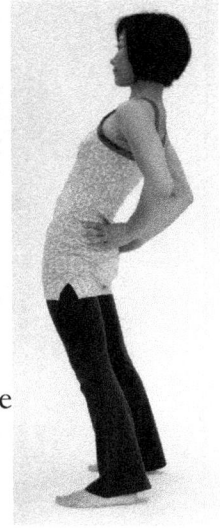

6.

Lower Back 2
HOGUSHI Massage

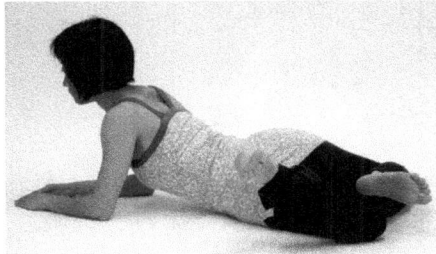

7. Lower Back 3
HOGUSHI Massage

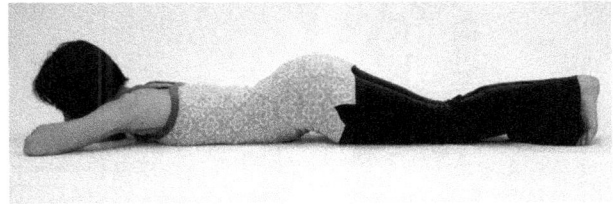

8. Lower Back 4
HOGUSHI Massage

9. Cobra Pose

Lie on the stomach, place the palms under the shoulders and lift the torso up, looking to the horizon.

Point

As it is a pose to bend backward, it is easier to do this pose after releasing the neck, shoulders and lower back. (Keep the hips on the ground.)

AFTER THE POSE

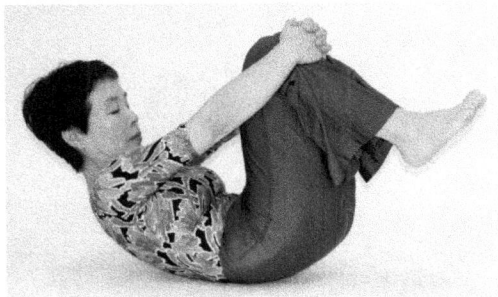

1. Lower Back 2
Counter Balance (p52)

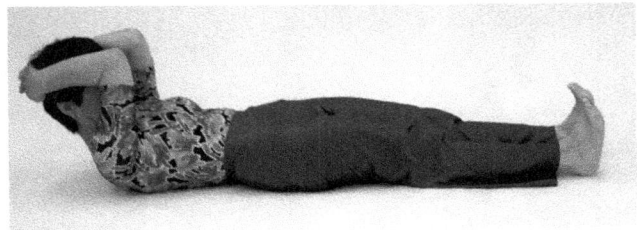

2. Neck 2 Counter Balance (p54)

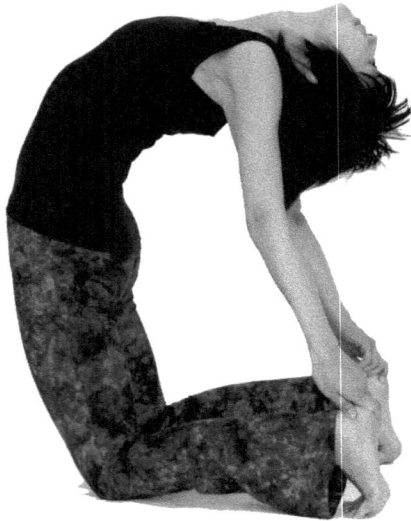

Camel

Effect: Releases stiffness in the shoulders. Builds up the strength of the heart and lungs. Increases flexibility in the neck, shoulder blades, arms and the lower back.

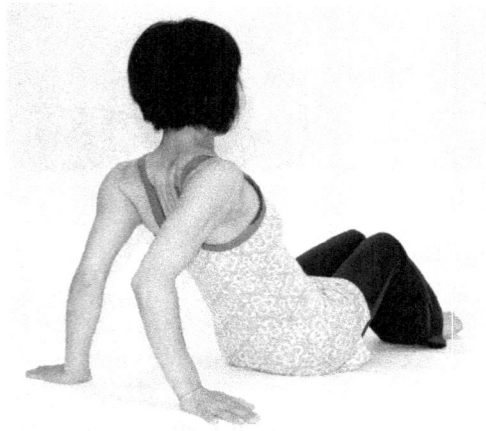

1. Shoulder Blades 1
   HOGUSHI Massage (p48)

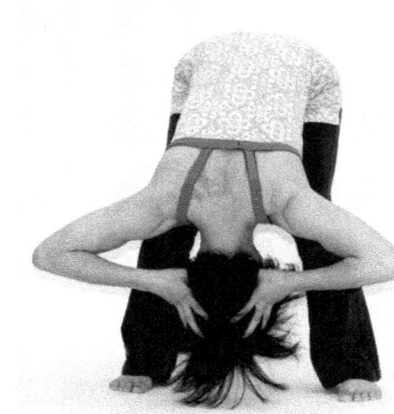

2. Neck and back of the Head 1
   HOGUSHI Massage (p50)

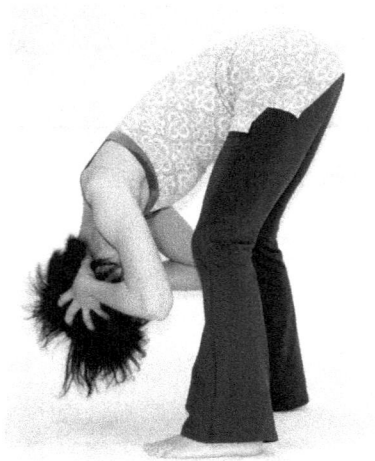

3. Neck and back of the Head 2
   HOGUSHI Massage

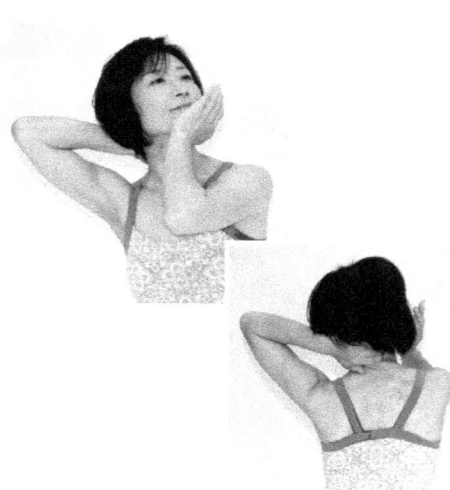

4. Neck and back of the Head 3
   HOGUSHI Massage

5.
Lower Back 1
HOGUSHI Massage
(p47)

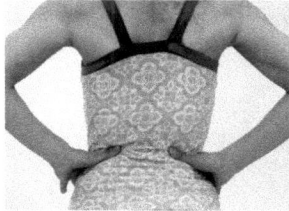

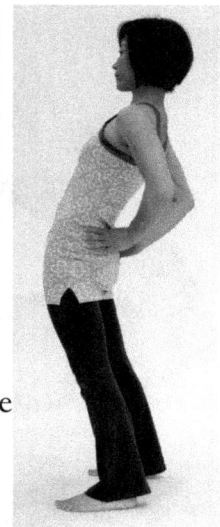

6.
Lower Back 2
HOGUSHI Massage

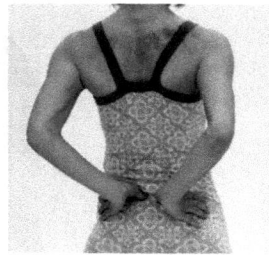

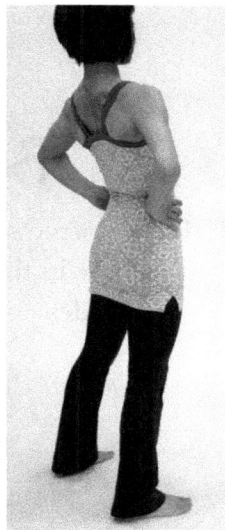

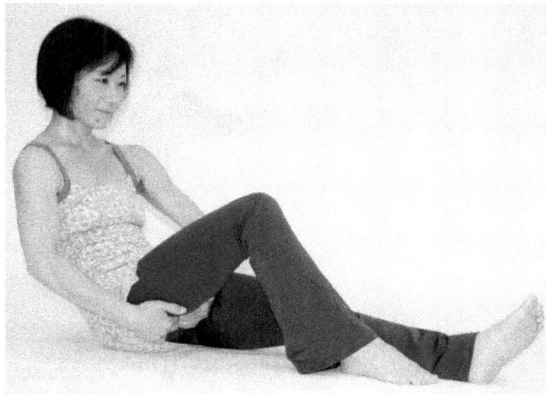

7. Legs 1 HOGUSHI Massage (p43)

8. Camel Pose

In an upright kneeling position, tuck the toes under, tuck the pelvis in. Place both hands on the ankles, lift the chest and open the chin to the sky.

Point
As it is a Back Bend pose, it is easier to do after releasing the neck, shoulders and the lower back.

AFTER THE POSE

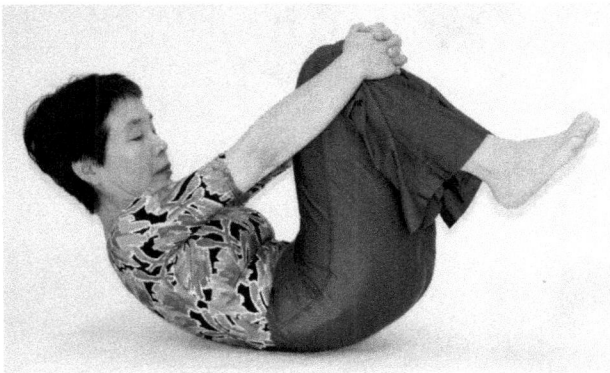

1. Lower Back 2
Counter Balance (p52)

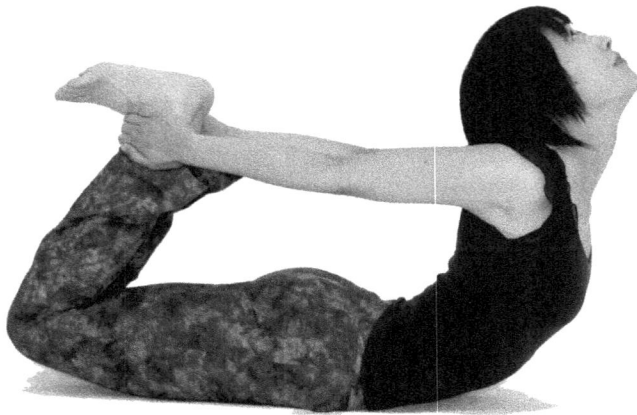

Bow

Effect: Corrects posture. Increases flexibility in the neck, shoulder blades and the arms.

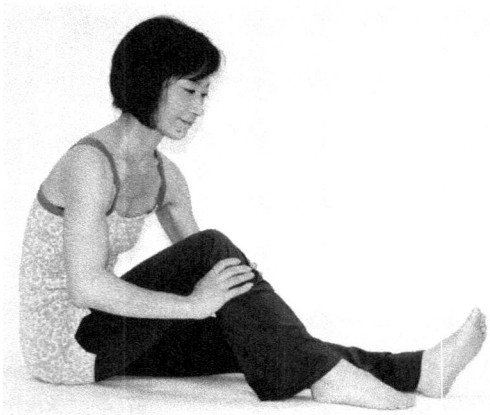

1. Legs 2 HOGUSHI Massage (p43)

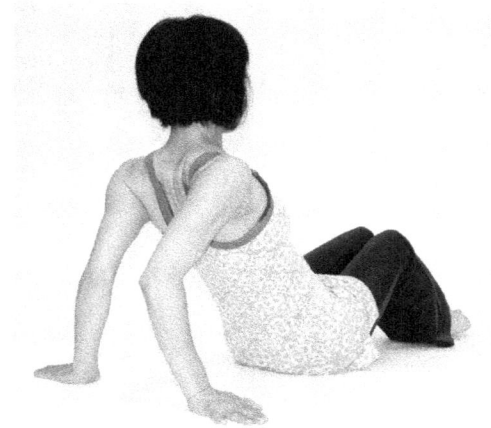

2. Shoulder Blades 1 HOGUSHI Massage (p48)

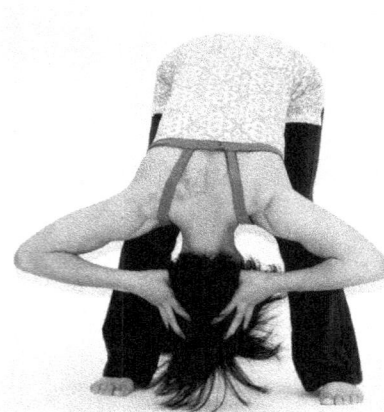

3. Neck and back of the Head 1 HOGUSHI Massage (p50)

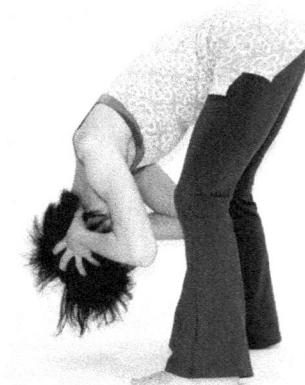

4. Neck and back of the Head 2 HOGUSHI Massage

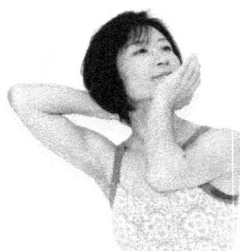

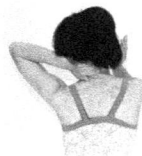

5. Neck and back of the Head 3 HOGUSHI Massage

Part 3 Releasing your body with HOGUSHI Massage

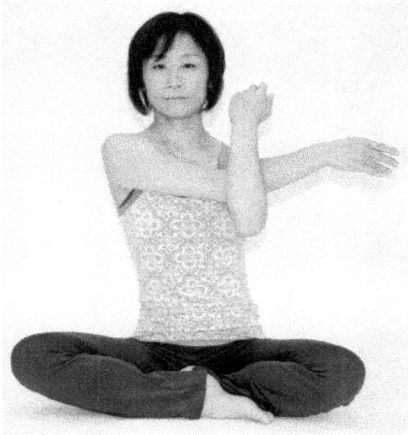

6. Shoulder Blades 2
HOGUSHI Massage (p48)

7. Lower Back 1
HOGUSHI Massage
(p47)

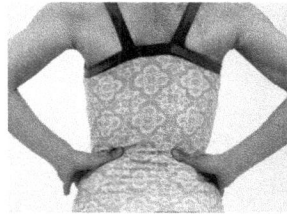

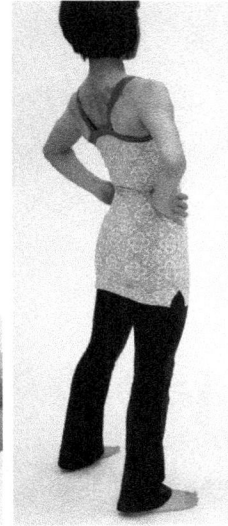

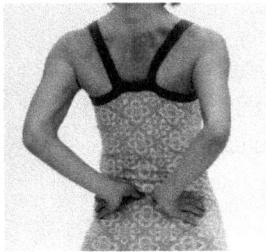

8. Lower Back 2
HOGUSHI Massage

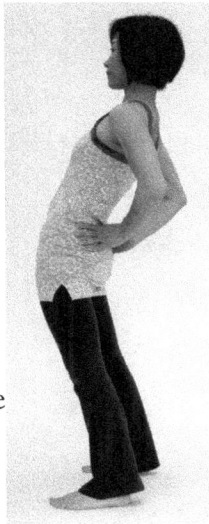

9. Bow Pose

Lie on the stomach, place the forehead on the ground, bend the knees and grab the ankles. Lift the thighs and chest off the ground and open the chin to stretch the front of the neck.

Point

As it is a Back Bend pose, it is easier to do this pose after releasing the neck, lower back and especially the shoulder blades.

AFTER THE POSE

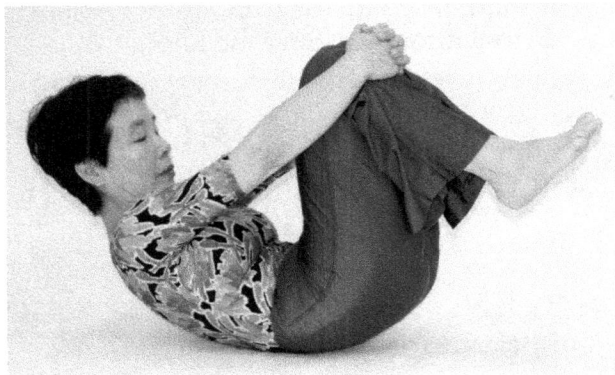

1. Lower Back 2
Counter Balance (p52)

Locust

Effect: Builds up the strength of the back muscles, lungs and the heart.

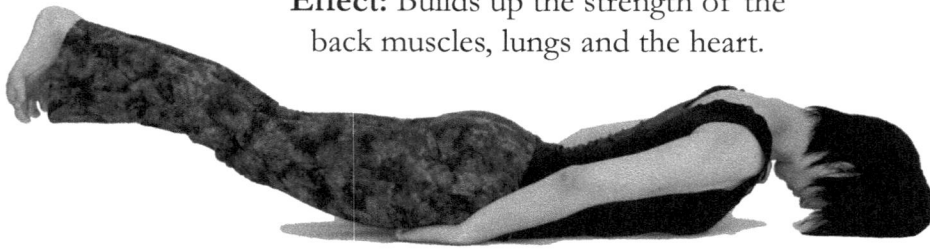

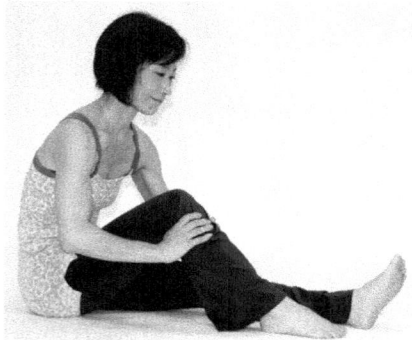

1. Legs 2 HOGUSHI Massage (p43)

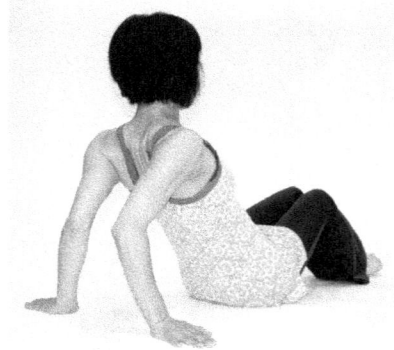

2. Shoulder Blades 1 HOGUSHI Massage (p48)

3.

Lower Back 1 HOGUSHI Massage (p47)

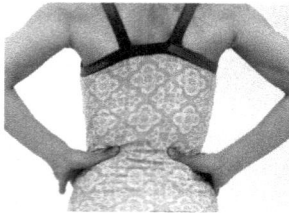

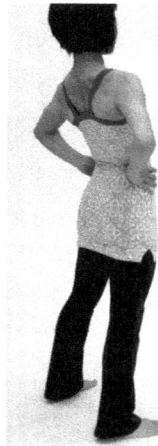

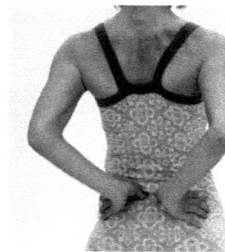

4.

Lower Back 2 HOGUSHI Massage

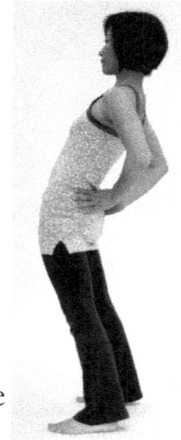

5. Locust Pose

Lie on the stomach with the forehead on the ground, place the fists under the base of the thighs, keep the ankles together and raise them without bending the knees while pressing the fists to the ground.

AFTER THE POSE

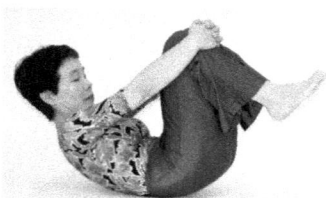

Point

As it is difficult for people with stiff back muscles to raise the legs, it is easier to do this pose after releasing the shoulder blades and lower back.

1. Lower Back 2 Counter Balance (p52)

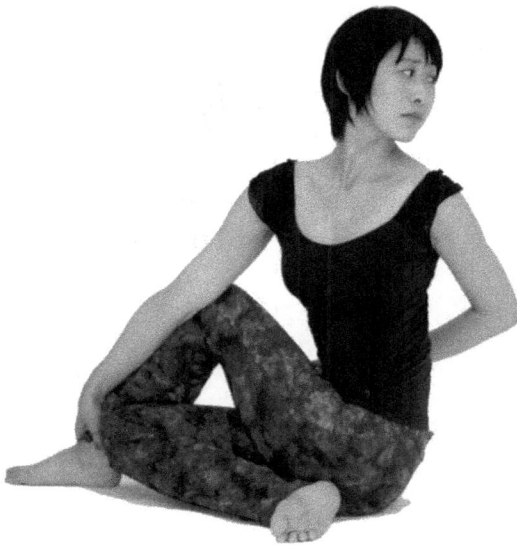

Twist

Effect: Corrects the upper body alignment. Removes fatigue. Increases flexibility in the shoulder blades and the lumber vertebrae.

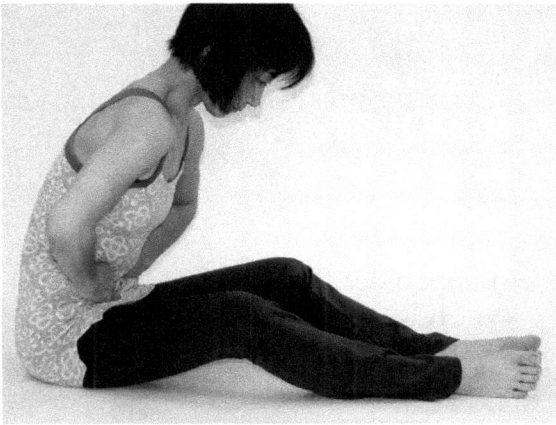

1. Abdomen 1HOGUSHI Massage (p46)

Point
It is difficult to twist the body when the torso is stiff, so twist the torso gently.

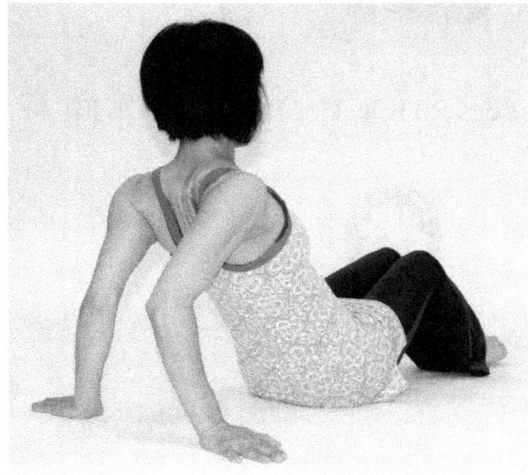

2. Shoulder Blades 1 HOGUSHI Massage (p48)

3. Twist Pose

In a seated position with straight legs, cross the legs, left leg over the right leg. Place the right arm along the lower left leg, grasping with the hand as low as possible. Twist the body to the left, while pressing the right elbow to left knee to perform stretch. Place the left arm behind the back to open the chest.

Repeat in opposite positions to the other side.

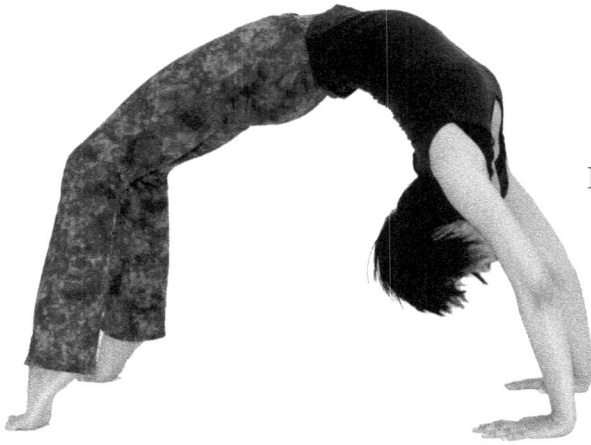

Bridge

Effect: Recovery from fatigue. Increases flexibility in the shoulder blades, back and the arms.

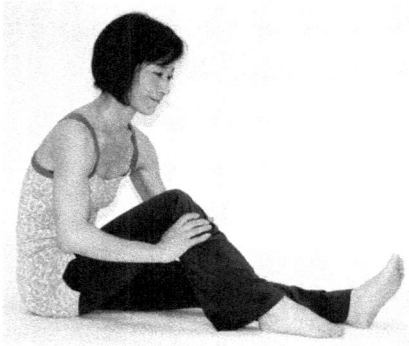

1. Legs 2 HOGUSHI Massage (p43)

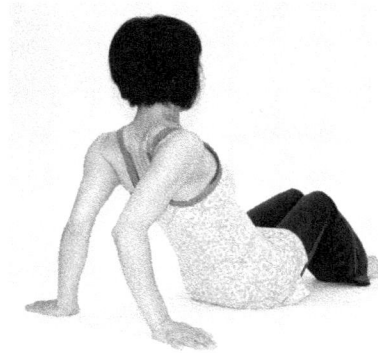

2. Shoulder Blades 1 HOGUSHI Massage (p48-49)

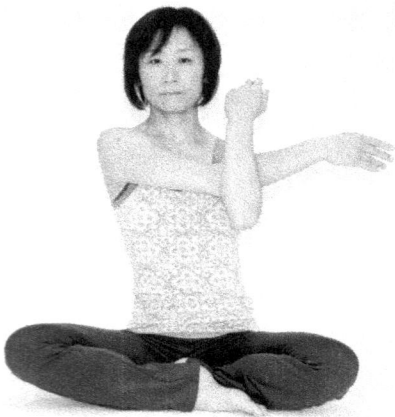

3. Shoulder Blades 2 HOGUSHI Massage

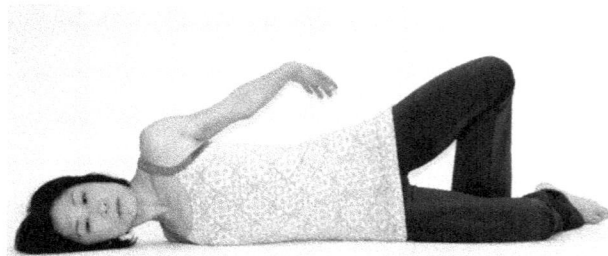

4. Shoulder Blades 3 HOGUSHI Massage

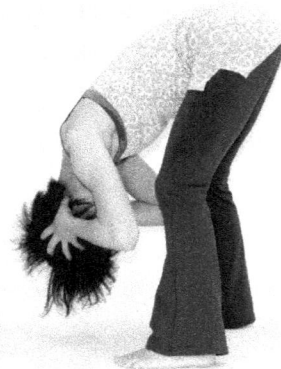

5. Neck and back of the Head 2 HOGUSHI Massage (p50)

Part 3 Releasing your body with HOGUSHI Massage

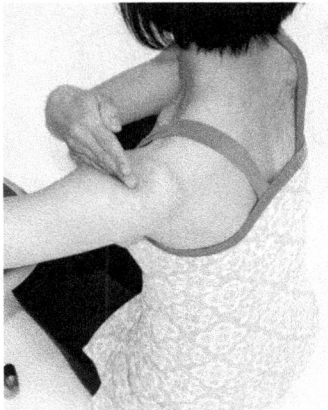

6. Shoulders and Arms 2
HOGUSHI Massage (p51)

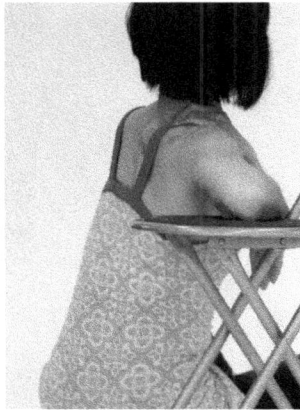

7. Shoulders and Arms 3
HOGUSHI Massage

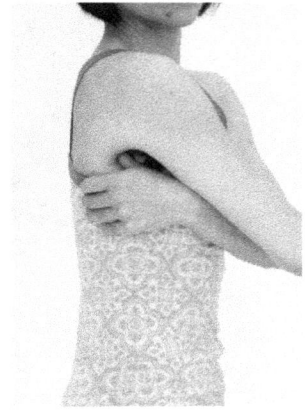

8. Shoulders and Arms 4
HOGUSHI Massage

9.

Lower Back 1
HOGUSHI Massage
(p47)

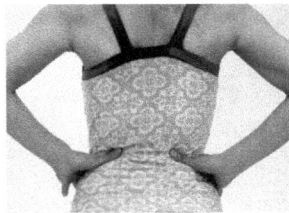

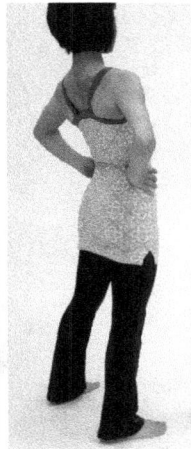

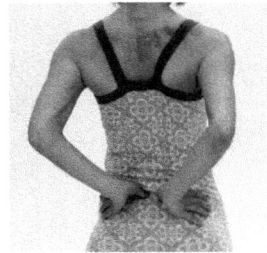

10.

Lower Back 2
HOGUSHI Massage

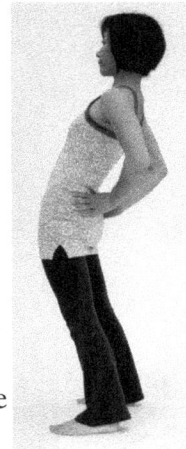

11. Lower Back 4
HOGUSHI Massage

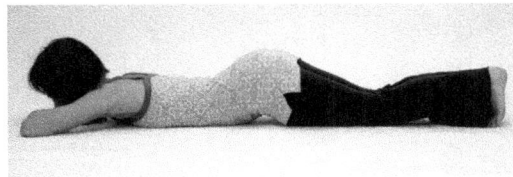

12. Bridge Pose

Lie on the back, bend the knees to place the heels close to the hips, place the palms beside the ears with fingers facing towards the shoulders. Lift the torso and raise the hips to the sky, (raise the heels off the ground), straighten the knees as much as possible and open the chest to the sky.

AFTER THE POSE

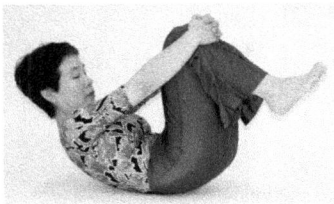

1. Lower Back 2
Counter Balance (p52)

Point

As it is a Back Bend pose, it is easier to do after releasing the shoulder blades, neck and lower back. Also, to straighten the arms in the pose, the shoulders and arms need to be released.

3 typical reasons that make it difficult to do this pose:
1. Stiff shoulder blades
2. Stiff lower back
3. The combination of stiff shoulder blades and lower back

Ensure that you carefully apply HOGUSHI Massage, particularly on the above areas.

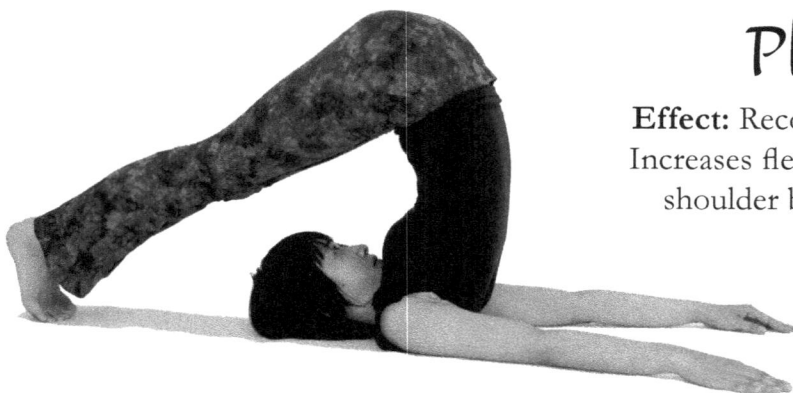

Plough

Effect: Recovery from fatigue. Increases flexibility in the neck, shoulder blades and torso.

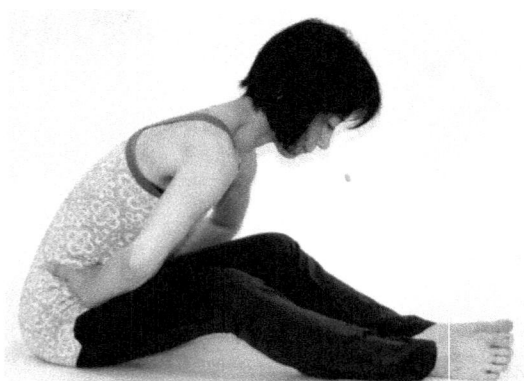

1. Abdomen 2
   HOGUSHI Massage (p46)

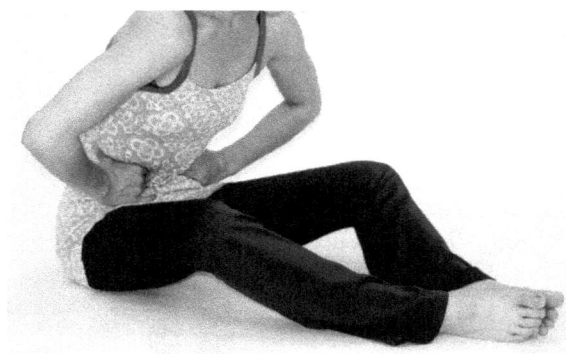

2. Abdomen 3
   HOGUSHI Massage

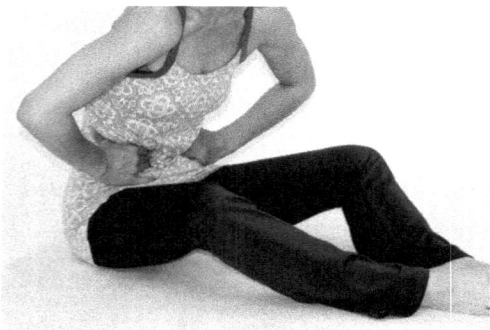

3. Abdomen 4
   HOGUSHI Massage

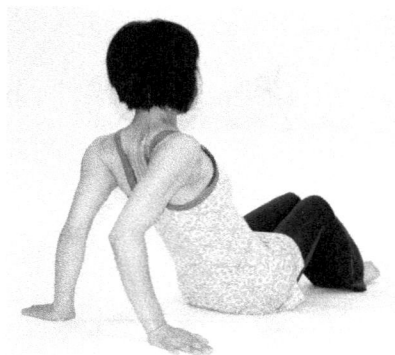

4. Shoulder Blades 1
   HOGUSHI Massage (p48)

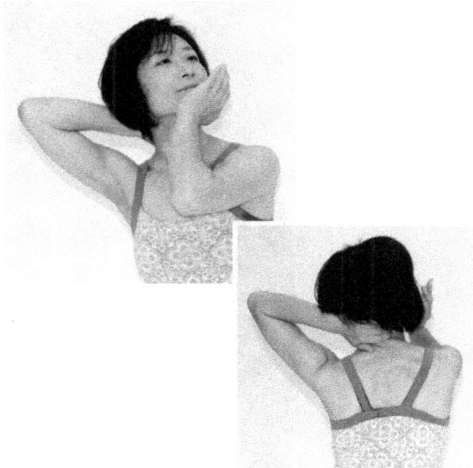

5. Neck and back of the Head 3
   HOGUSHI Massage (p50)

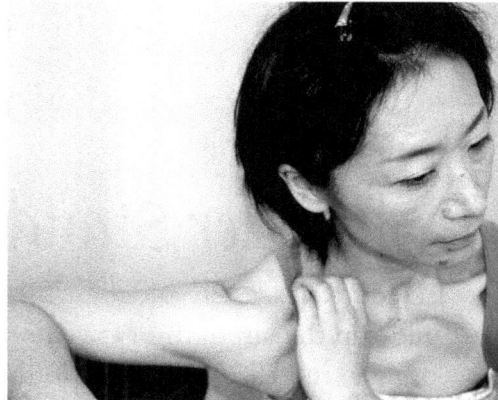

6. Shoulders and Arms 1
   HOGUSHI Massage (p51)

7. Plough Pose

Lie on the back, place the palms on the ground beside the body. Raise the legs vertically to the sky and then drop them over towards the head to place the toes on the ground.

Point

As this pose curls the body, it is important to release the abdomen, shoulder blades and the neck.

AFTER THE POSE

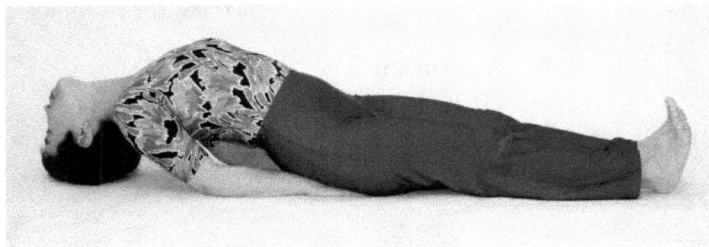

1. Neck 1
   Counter Balance (p54)

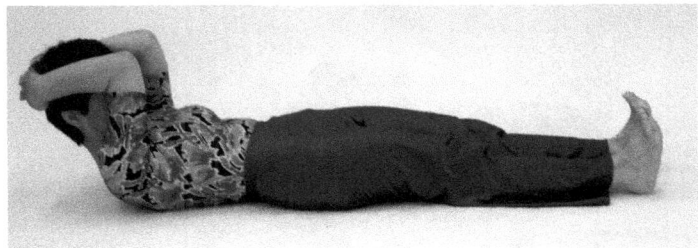

2. Neck 2
   Counter Balance

Shoulder Stand

Effect: Releases shoulder stiffness. Builds up the strength in the internal organs. Increases flexibility in the neck and the shoulder blades.

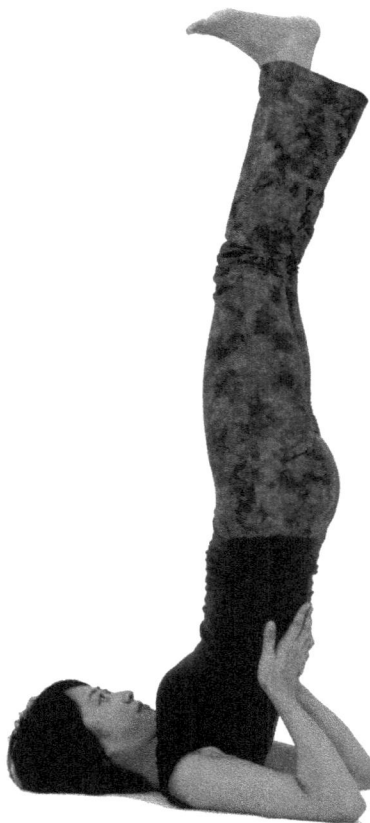

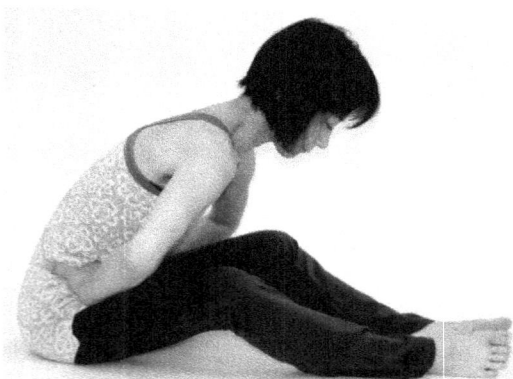

1. Abdomen 2
HOGUSHI Massage (p46)

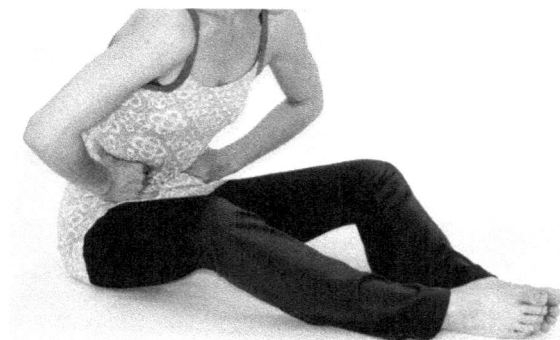

2. Abdomen 3
HOGUSHI Massage

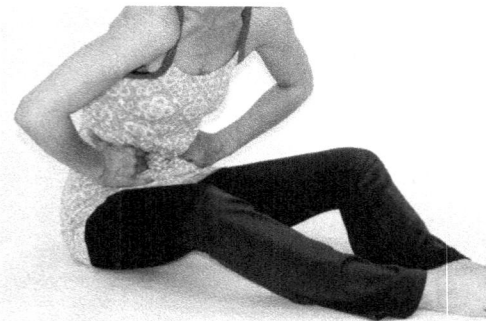

3. Abdomen 4
HOGUSHI Massage

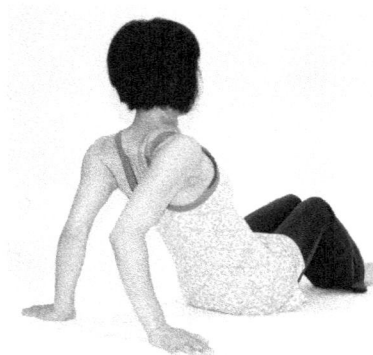

4. Shoulder Blades 1
HOGUSHI Massage (p48)

Part 3   Releasing your body with HOGUSHI Massage

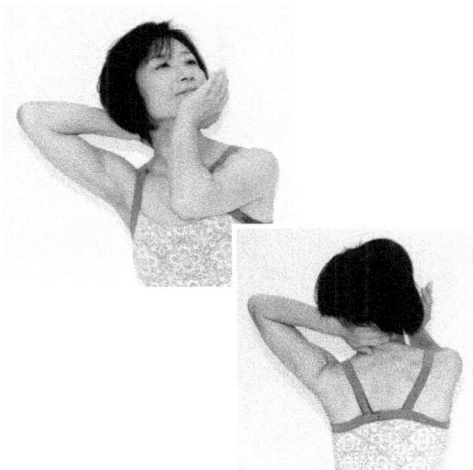

$5.$ Neck and back of the Head 3
HOGUSHI Massage (p50)

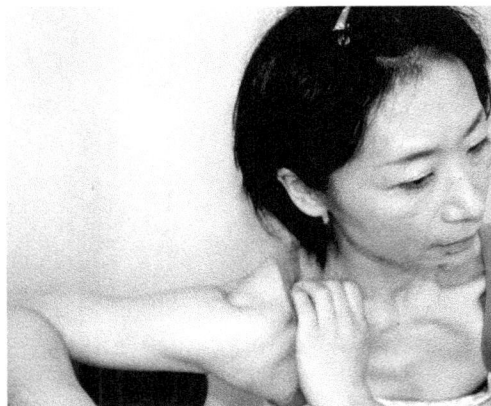

$6.$ Shoulders and Arms 1
HOGUSHI Massage (p51)

$7.$ Shoulder Stand

Lie on the back, arms beside body, palms down. Raise the legs vertically to the sky and flex the ankles to make the soles of the feet parallel to the ground. Bend the knees a little and lift pelvis and torso off the ground, bracing the elbows into the ground and placing the hands on the lower back to support, straighten the knees and raise the legs to a vertical position.

Point

It is important to release the abdomen, neck and especially the shoulder blades, as this helps to place the elbows closer together on the ground to stabilise and support the body while being inverted.

AFTER THE POSE

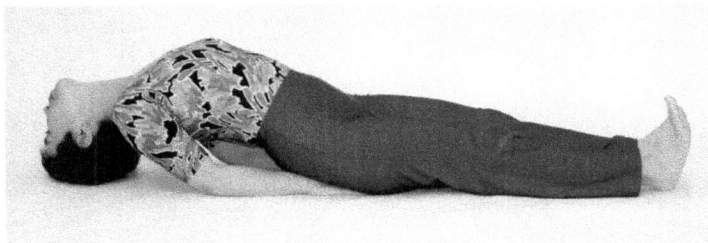

$1.$ Neck 1
Counter Balance (p54)

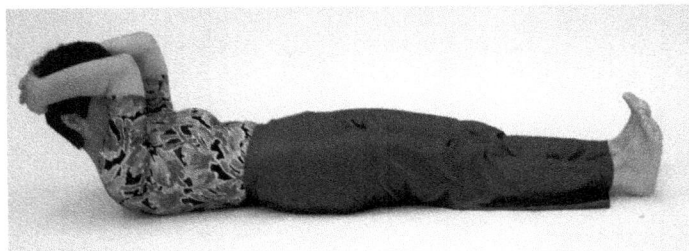

$2.$ Neck 2
Counter Balance

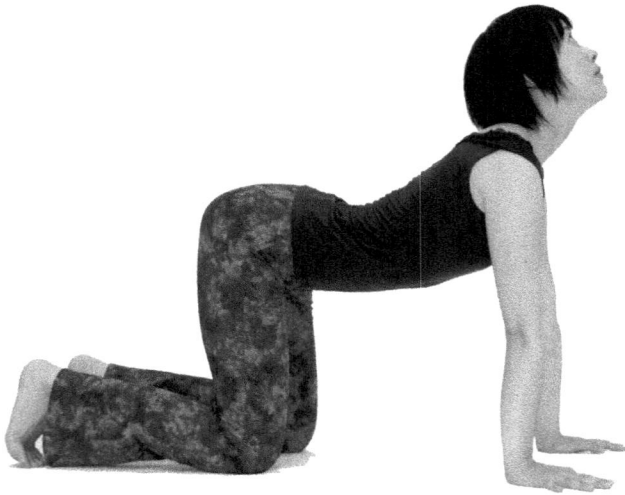

Cat

Effect: Increases flexibility in the back.

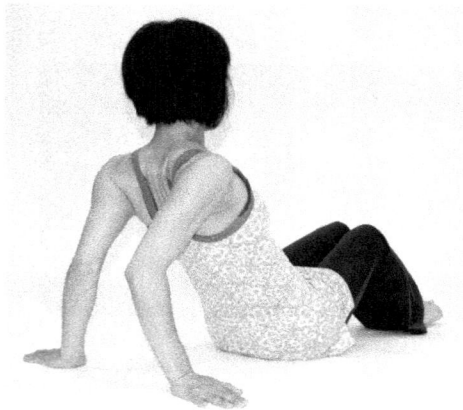

1. Shoulder Blades 1
   HOGUSHI Massage (p48)

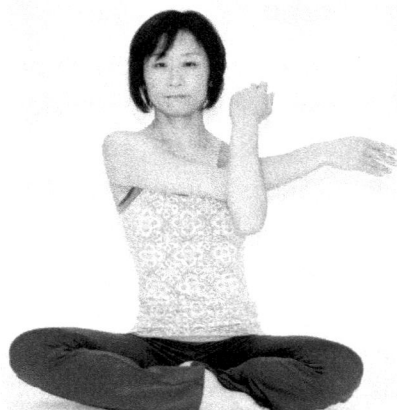

2. Shoulder Blades 2
   HOGUSHI Massage

It is easier to do Cat Pose after massaging the neck

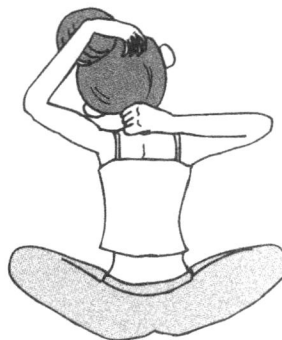

3.

Lower Back 1
HOGUSHI Massage
(p47)

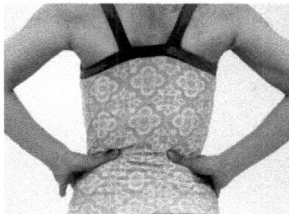

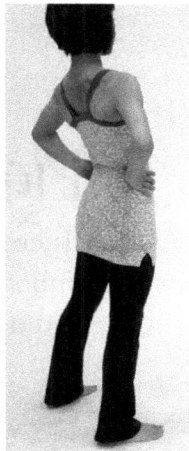

4.

Lower Back 4
HOGUSHI Massage

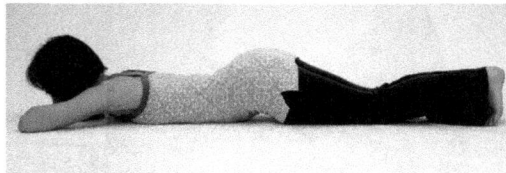

5. Cat Pose

In an all fours position with legs waist width apart, open the chin and arch the spine, looking up.

Point
Massage the shoulder blades, lower back and the neck well.

AFTER THE POSE

1.

Lower Back 4
Counter Balance (p53)

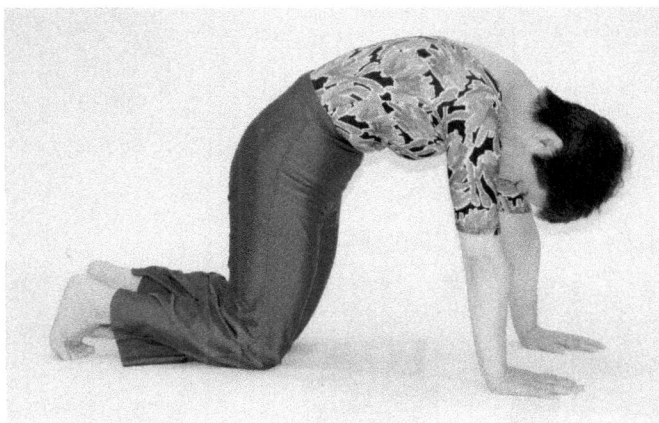

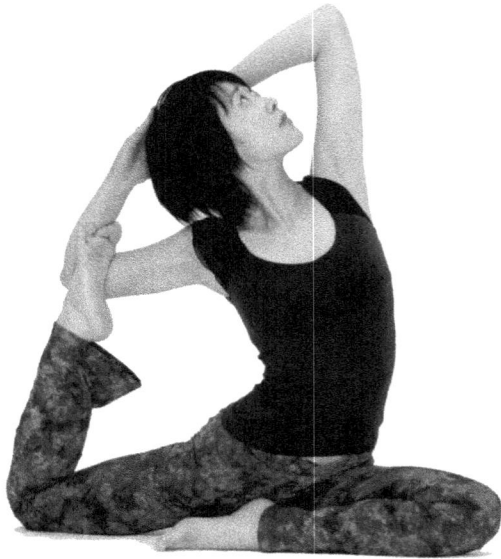

Pigeon

Effect: Increases flexibility in the lumbar vertebrae and the legs.

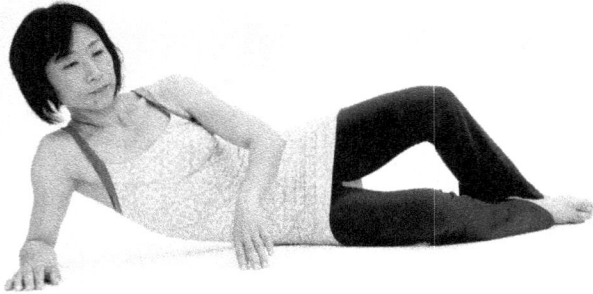

1. Hips 4
   HOGUSHI Massage (p41)

2. Hips 5
   HOGUSHI Massage

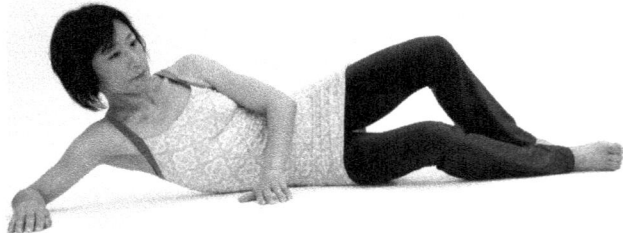

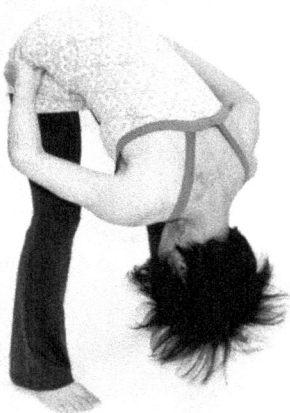

3. Groin Area 2
   HOGUSHI Massage (p44)

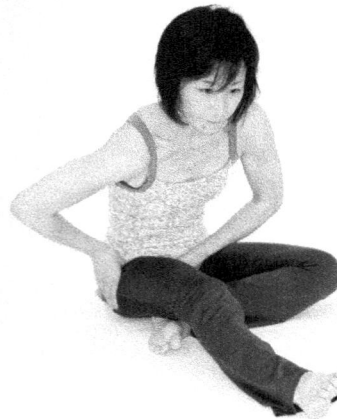

4. Groin Area 3
   HOGUSHI Massage

Part 3 Releasing your body with HOGUSHI Massage

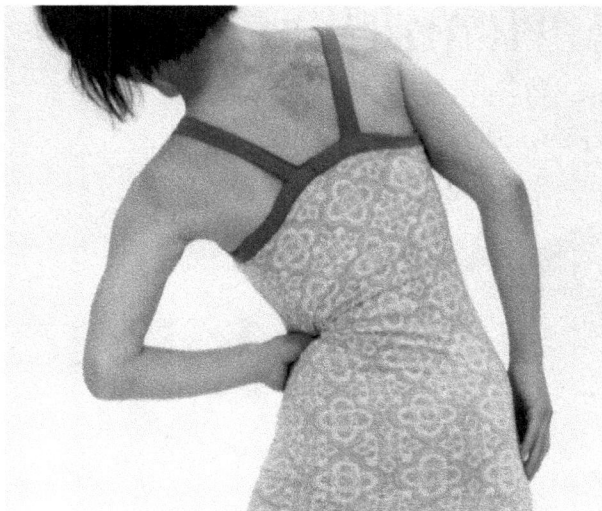

5.
Side of the Torso 1
HOGUSHI Massage
(p45)

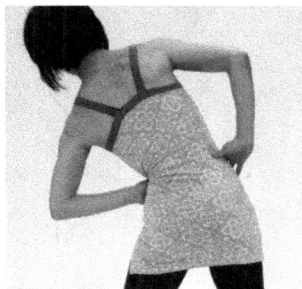

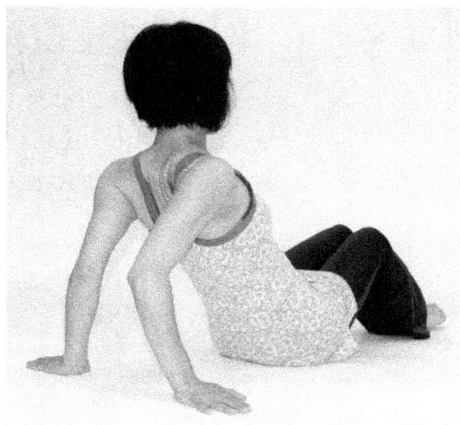

6. Shoulder Blades 1
HOGUSHI Massage (p48)

7. Pigeon Pose

Sit with the legs bent in front and draw the right leg back – place the hip to the ground as close as possible. Bend the right knee up and hook the toes by the right elbow area. Place the hands behind the head and clasp fingers. Raise the left arm and pull the elbow further back, bend the right elbow to grasp fingers. Repeat on the other side.

Point
Before doing this pose, it is best to massage well on the hip and groin areas. This pose is made easier by doing Twist Pose beforehand.

AFTER THE POSE

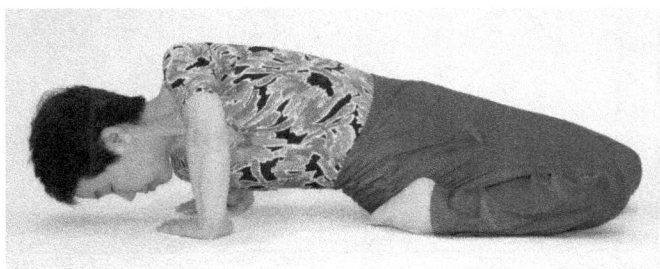

1. Lower Back 3
Counter Balance (p53)

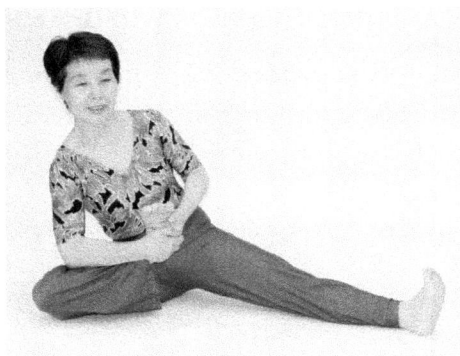

2. Knees 1
Counter Balance (p54)

Open Legged Forward Bend

Effect: Reduces swelling and circulation in the legs by improving blood flow in the lower abdominal area. Recovery from fatigue in the legs. Increases flexibility in the inner thighs.

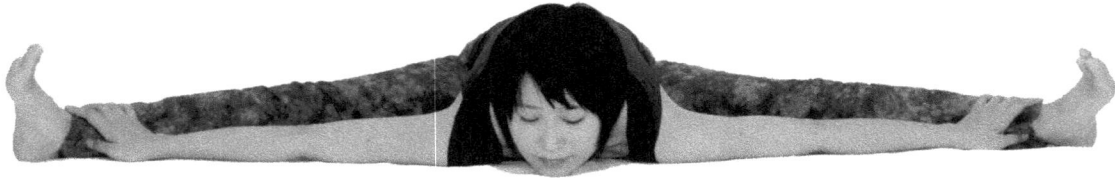

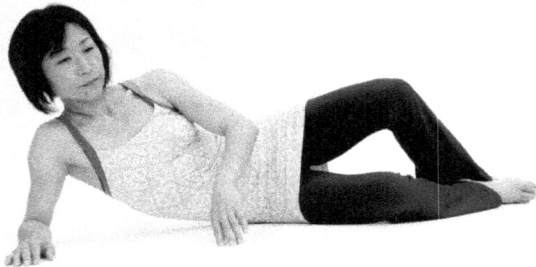

1. Hips 4
   HOGUSHI Massage (p41-42)

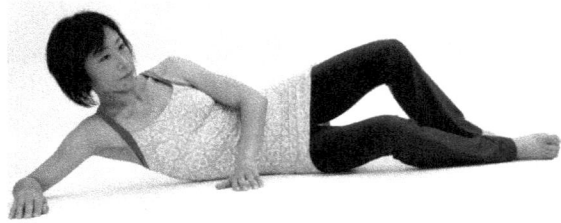

2. Hips 5
   HOGUSHI Massage

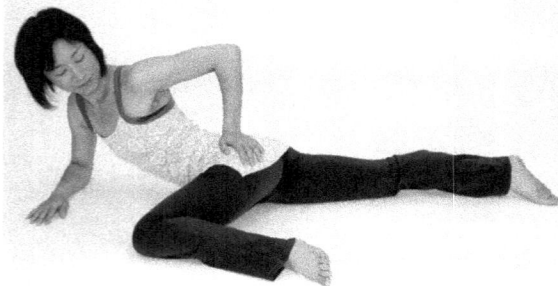

3. Hips 6
   HOGUSHI Massage

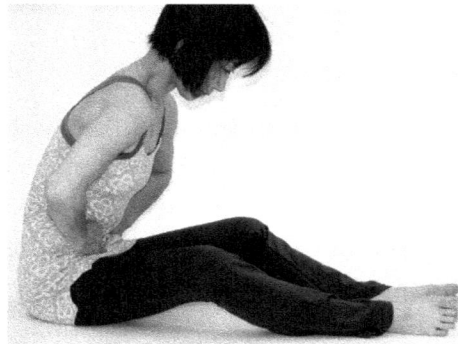

4. Abdomen 1
   HOGUSHI Massage (p46)

5. **Open Legs Forward Bend**

Sit on the ground and spread the legs wide in an open legged position. Bend forward with the aim to touch the chest to the ground.

Point

To reduce any pain and make it easier to perform, shake and massage the muscles around the pubic bone while doing the pose.

AFTER THE POSE

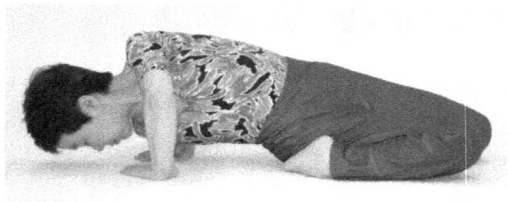

1. Lower Back 3
   Counter Balance (p53)

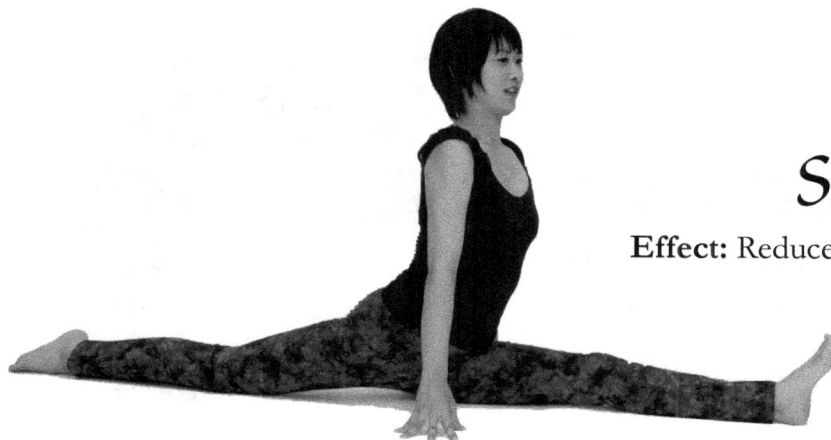

Splits

Effect: Reduces swelling in the legs.

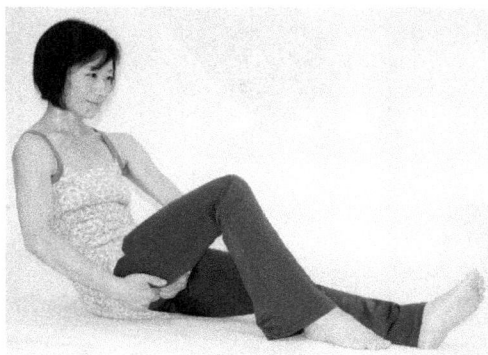

1. Legs 1 HOGUSHI Massage (p43)

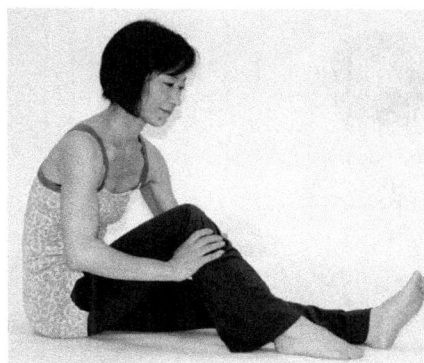

2. Legs 2 HOGUSHI Massage

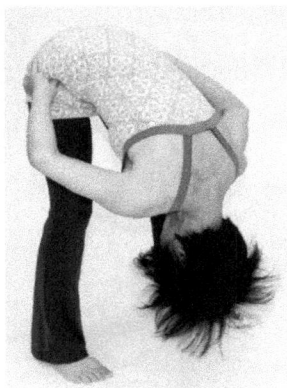

3. Groin Area 2 HOGUSHI Massage (p44)

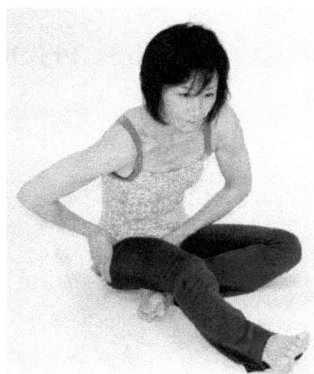

4. Groin Area 3 HOGUSHI Massage

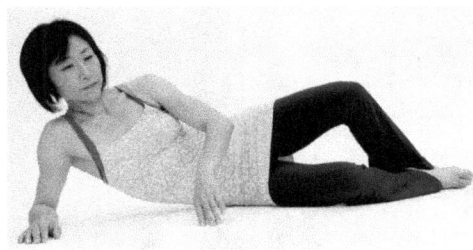

5. Hips 4 HOGUSHI Massage (p41)

6. Splits

Split the legs forward and backward. Repeat on the other side.

Point

It is easier to do this pose by massaging well the muscles around the back of the ilium, between the hips and legs.

Standing Back Bend

Effect: Corrects posture. Increases flexibility in the neck, shoulder blades and spine.

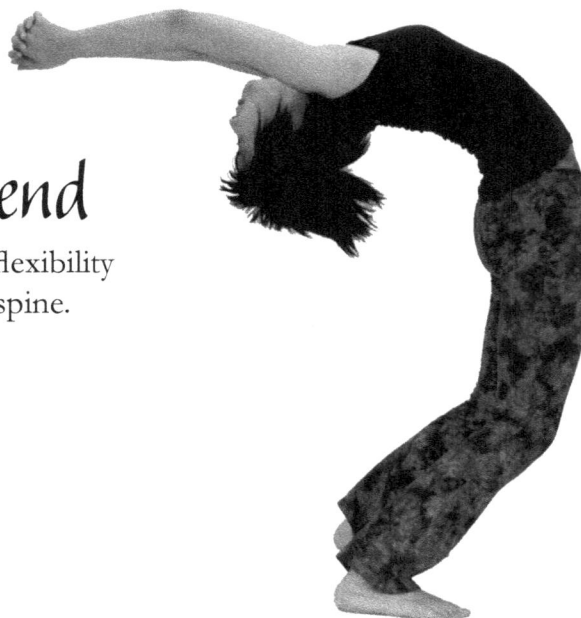

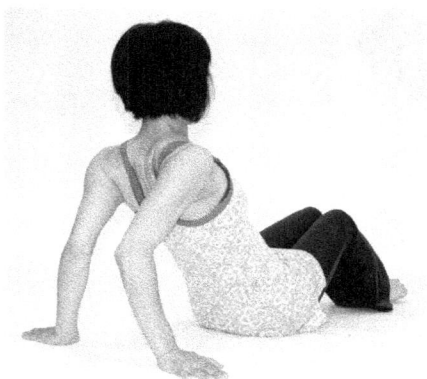

1. Shoulder Blades 1
HOGUSHI Massage (p48)

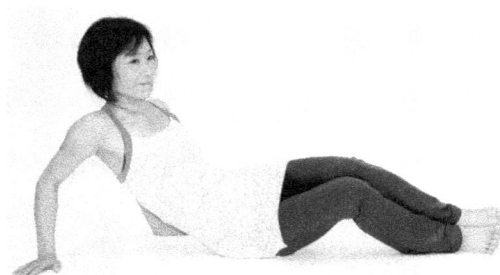

2. Hips 2 HOGUSHI Massage (p40)

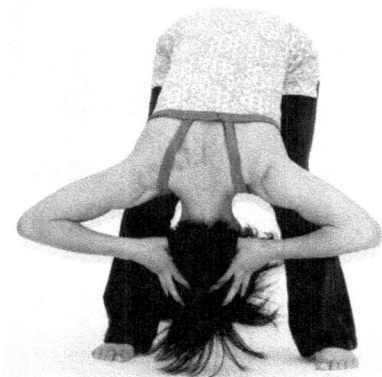

3.
Neck and Back of the Head 1
HOGUSHI Massage (p50)

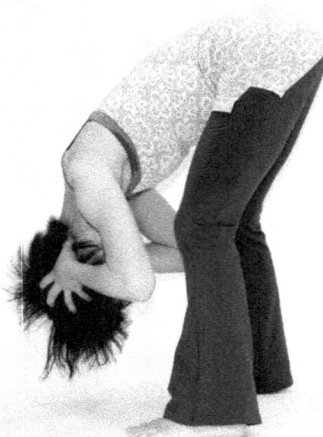

4.
Neck and Back of the Head 2
HOGUSHI Massage

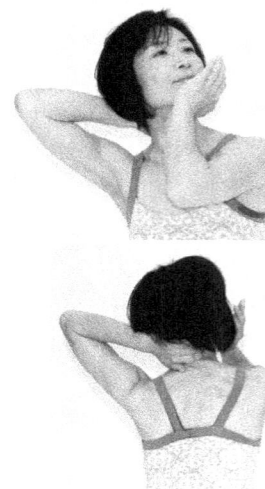

5.
Neck and back of the Head 3
HOGUSHI Massage

6.
Shoulders & Arms 3
HOGUSHI Massage
(p51)

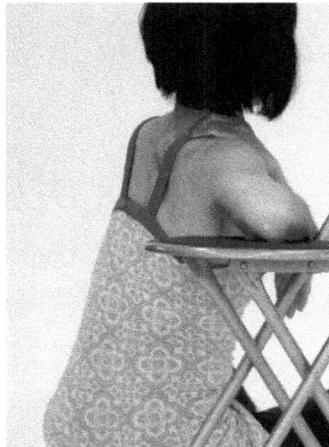

7.
Lower Back 1
HOGUSHI Massage
(p47)

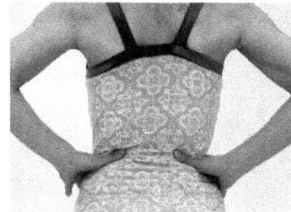

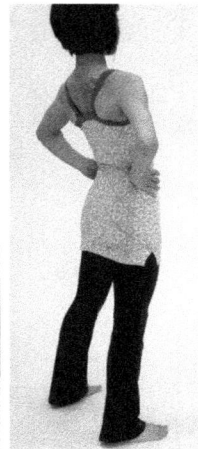

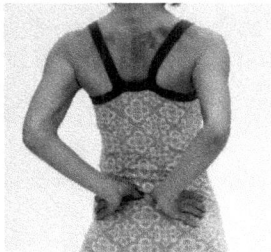

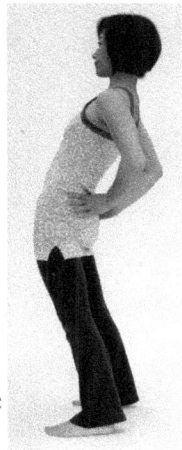

8.
Lower Back 2
HOGUSHI Massage

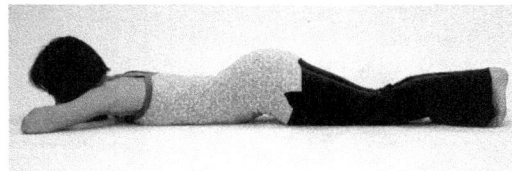

9.
Lower Back 4
HOGUSHI Massage

10. **Standing Back Bend**

In the standing position, bend the upper body over.

Point
Before doing this pose, massage the neck, shoulder blades and the torso sides to release the lower back area well.

AFTER THE POSE

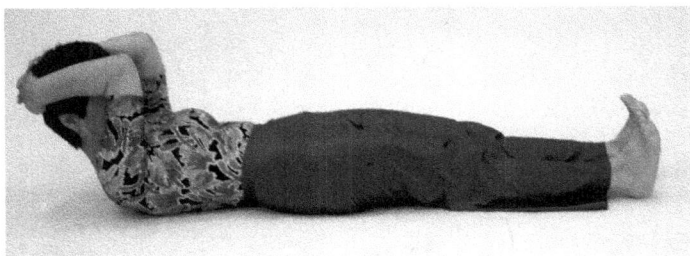

1.
Neck 2
Counter Balance (p54)

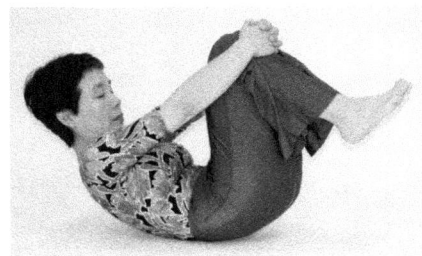

2.
Lower Back 2
Counter Balance (p52)

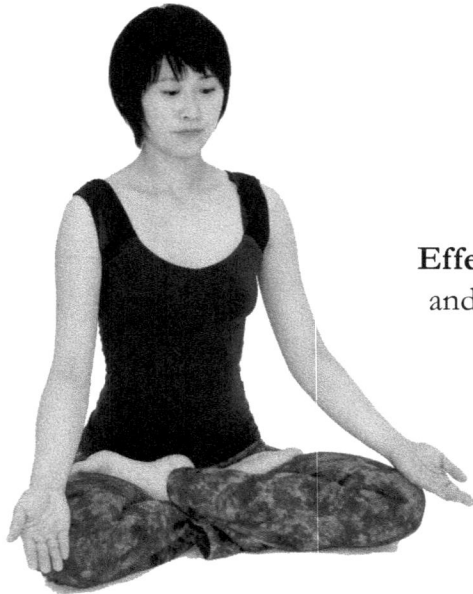

Lotus

Effect: Increases flexibility in the hip joints and knees by improving blood flow in the lower abdominal area and the legs.

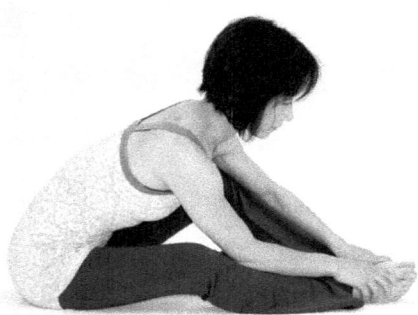

$1.$ Hips 1 HOGUSHI Massage (p40-41)

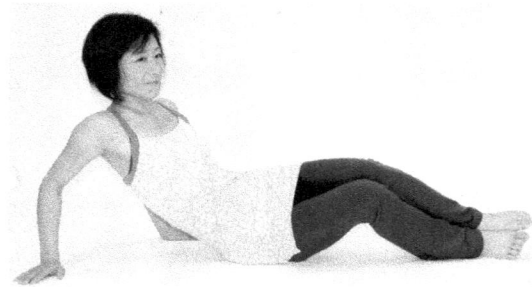

$2.$ Hips 2 HOGUSHI Massage

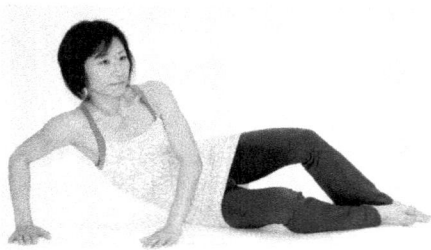

$3.$ Hips 3 HOGUSHI Massage

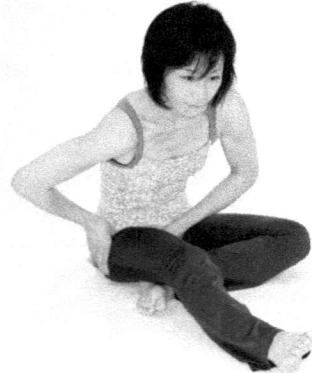

$4.$ Groin Area 1 HOGUSHI Massage (p44)

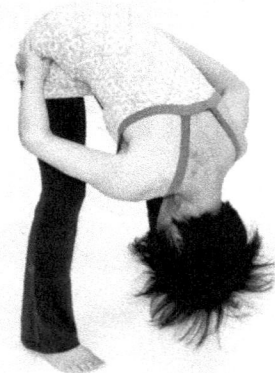

$5.$ Groin Area 2 HOGUSHI Massage

AFTER THE POSE

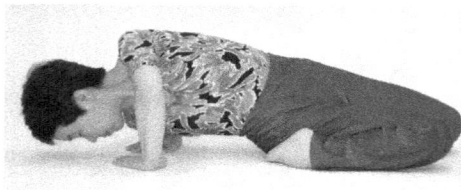

Point

By massaging on the front and back areas between the legs and the hips, it is easier to do this pose.

$1.$ Lower Back 3 Counter Balance (p53)

Part 3 Releasing your body with HOGUSHI Massage

Forward Bend in Butterfly

Effect: Increases flexibility in the hip joints and knees by improving blood flow in the lower abdominal area and the legs.

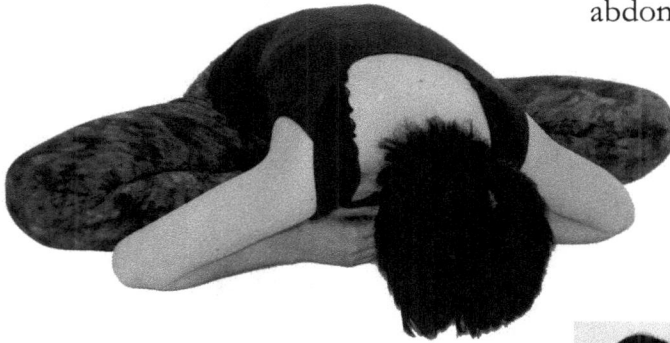

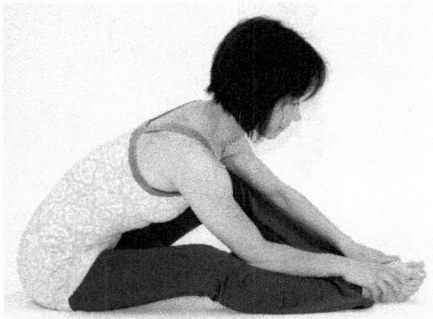

1. Hips 1 HOGUSHI Massage (p40)

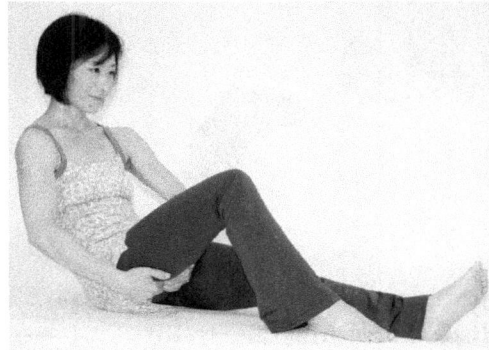

2. Legs 1 HOGUSHI Massage (p43)

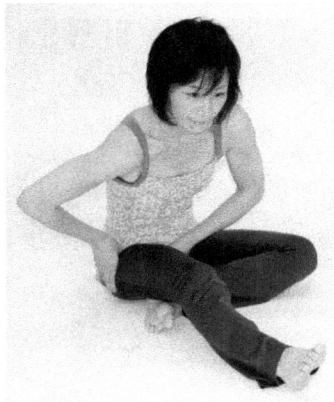

3. Groin Area 1 HOGUSHI Massage (p44)

4. Forward Bend in Butterfly Pose

Sit with bent knees with the soles of the feet touching together, grab the feet and bend forward from the lower back.

Point

Hips 1 and Groin Area 1 HOGUSHI Massage are effective for people having difficulty tucking the pelvis in.

AFTER THE POSE

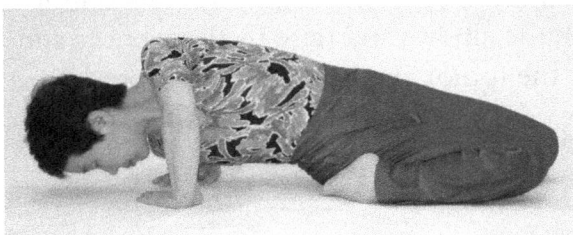

1. Lower Back 3 Counter Balance (p53)

Head Stand

Effect: Reduces shoulder stiffness and corrects body alignment.

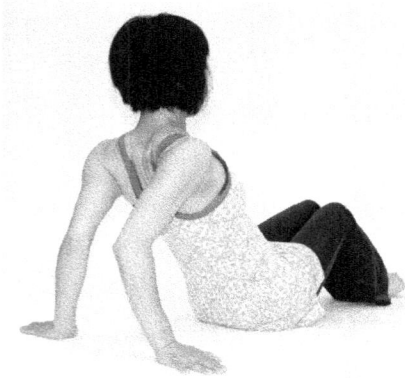

1. Shoulder Blades 1
   HOGUSHI Massage (p48)

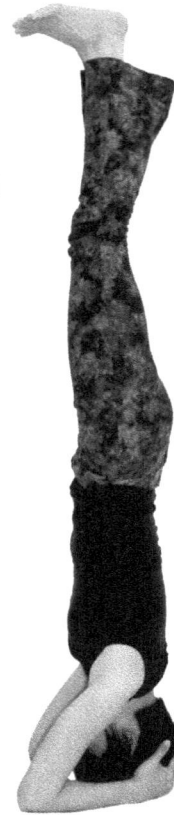

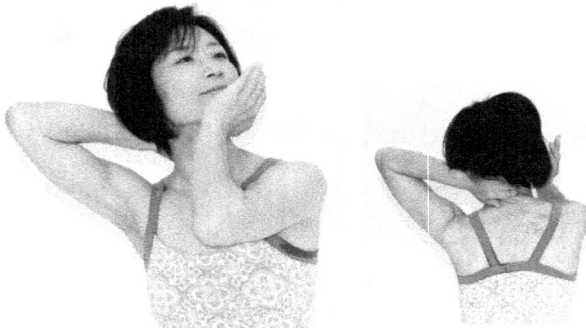

2. Neck and back of the Head 3
   HOGUSHI Massage (p50)

Point

It is important to massage well on the shoulder blades and the neck as a stiff back tends to curl up and roll over when raising the legs.

3. Head Stand

In a kneeling position, interlace fingers, place the elbows on the ground in front. Place the top of the head on the ground inside the fingers, stretch the legs and walk on the toes towards the body. Support the body with the elbows and raise the legs, knees and ankles to the sky to form a straight line from the top of the head to the bottom of the heels.

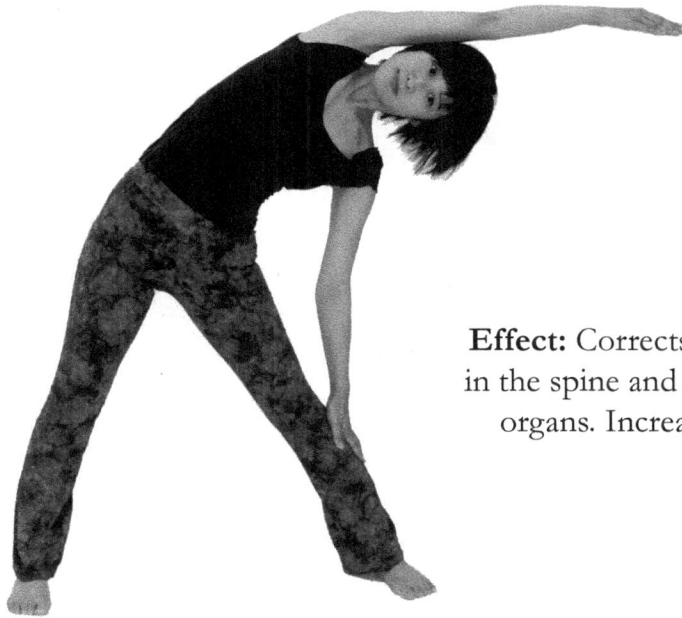

Hook

Effect: Corrects posture. Builds up strength in the spine and the functions of the internal organs. Increases flexibility in the spine.

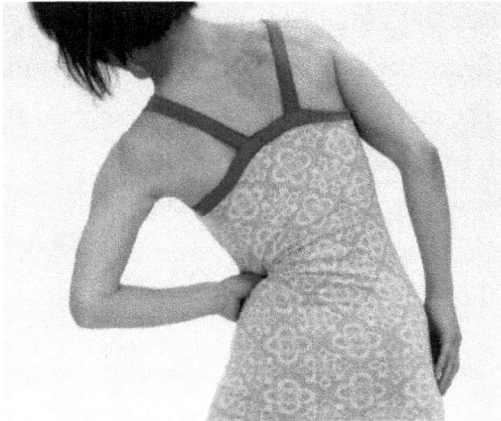

1. Side of the Torso 1
HOGUSHI Massage (p45)

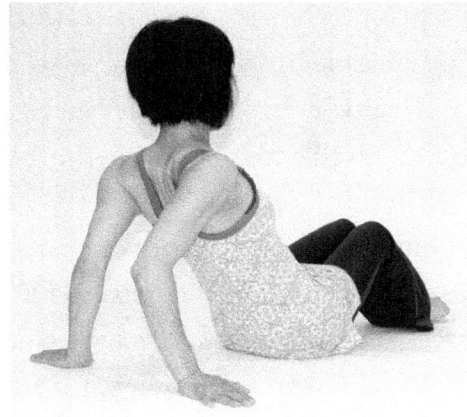

2. Shoulder Blades 1
HOGUSHI Massage (p48)

3. Hook Pose

Stand with your feet parallel to each other at shoulder width apart, stretch the arms out to the sides, drop the shoulders, slide the body to the left side as far as possible. Place the left arm on the side of left calf and stretch downward while touching the right arm to the right ear and stretching out, as far as possible.

AFTER THE POSE

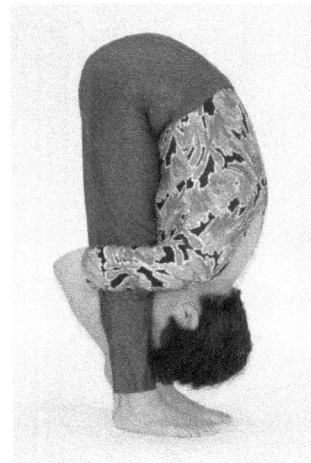

1.
Lower Back 5
Counter Balance
(p53)

Point
By applying finger pressure on the soft spots around the waist, it is easier to bend to the side.

Diet that helps soften the body

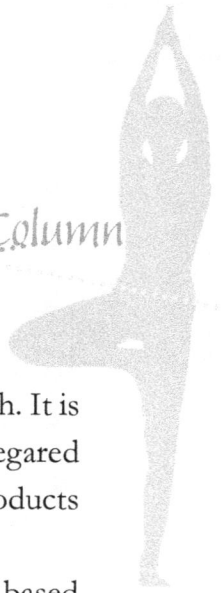

To soften the body, cut down on the intake of animal proteins such as meat and fish. It is recommended to have a more vegetable based diet and include some fruit and vinegared food. With stocks, try not to use chemical based seasonings but use natural products such as seaweeds and mushrooms.

To further increase flexibility, it would be necessary to continue a vegetable based diet for many years. Some people say that: "It has had no effect even though I have kept the diet for a week", or, "Nothing has changed even after a month". But remember, these people are already tight from eating an animal protein dominant diet over a long period of time. It is not possible to see any dramatic change in such a short period.

The bodies' metabolic temperature becomes slightly cooler with a vegetable based diet. Due to this, the ability of the immune system will drop a little.

When you feel the body getting cold, some weakness or acquired flexibility waning, then enjoy the achievements accomplished so far and have some animal protein. Of course, please avoid having excessive amounts. Do have well balanced meals!

NB. It is good to have a little animal protein in winter when the body requires some heat and less in summer when it is hotter.

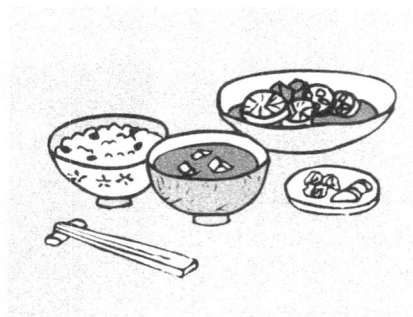

Part 4:
HOGUSHI Massage
for your heart

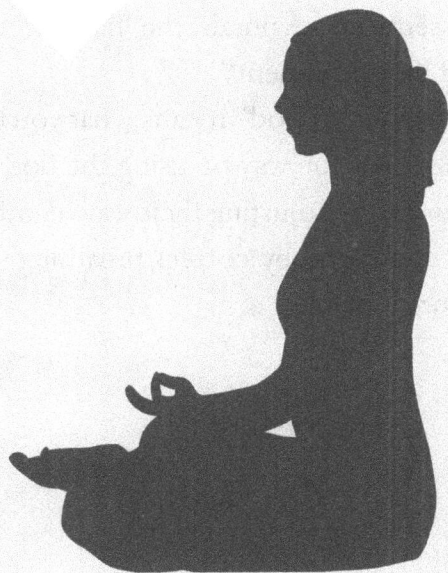

The more open the mind, the more flexible the body

When the mind is relaxed it is easier to soften the body. It's natural to be more relaxed and flexible after having a good time with friends.

As you can imagine, the mind has a significant effect on the body. The digestive organs are easily influenced by the mental status. According to experiments by American doctors, the stomach shrinks with congestion after being told negative things.

Additionally, people can have constipation due to mental stresses. Liver spots will easily appear on the cheeks when the liver becomes tight and it is difficult to get rid of them regardless of the effort applied to skin whitening.

It is hard to increase flexibility, no matter how much HOGUSHI Massage and stretching is being done, for people **who are suffering from regular stress, who are constant worrywarts, or who have a nervous temperament and/or meticulous nature.**

By cultivating an open mind and aiming to encompass a relaxed life style, the body can develop softness; it then becomes easier to further increase flexibility by HOGUSHI Massage and stretching. Ridding the cheeks of liver spots is then easier.

To maintain a relaxed life style, it is important to contemplate a balanced life. In yoga, five elements are considered as essential to maintain the 'balance' in human life; "Breath", "Food", "Idea", "Movement" and "Environment".

"Breath" means breathing technique, "Food" means what you ingest, "Idea" means the way of thinking and "Movement" means the way of using the body.

People are able to balance their life by adjusting their way of thinking in regards to their "Environment", such as at home and work, by correct breathing, having supportive food and moving the body (see the Figure 7 below).

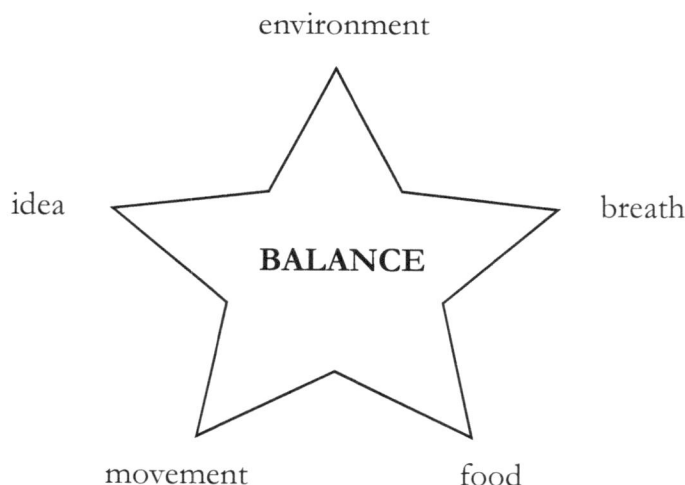

Figure 7

These five elements are linked with each other.

Having a bad posture in any physical movement creates shallow breathing. Under various environmental conditions, breathing is also changed.

Breath tends to be deeper at home or when having a good time with friends and is shallower under work stresses. By having excessive amounts of animal products and too much junk food, waste products and toxins stay within the body and it becomes blocked, stiff and flexibility is limited. Also, a consequence of a rigid body is a narrow mind.

Heart pains are a warning

My Oki-do Master taught me that "Life force is God", which ultimately, conveys the meaning to obey the 'teaching of the life force' to balance your life. When there is pain somewhere in the body while doing a yoga pose, it's a warning from the life force to do something to correct it.

This is the same with the mind.

It is an alert from the heart when there is mental suffering due to anxiety and stress, and a warning for something to be done about the current state. The heart is trying to say something is wrong in the way of thinking or concepts.

Under these conditions, there may be relief if the way of thinking can be changed. There are numerous things that we are unable to do the way we would like, be it in our own home or community.

Consider such behaviour as not responding to a letter from your spouse's mother because of dislike or not concentrating when a work superior is teaching a new task?

This might hurt their feelings and generate a grudge against such conduct. This can create more exposure to stress due to the potentially worse relationships with them.

Family and friends are important for everyone. So consider others when showing a displeased face or when disagreeable things are said to make others feel unpleasant. Even at work, superiors and co-workers will not communicate if shown a cold heart all the time. By listening honestly to what people have to say and by doing things in an amicable manner, work and relationships will become more congenial.

For people in the customer service industry, good results will come from work if customers are treated with respect and a frank and open attitude is held in response to their requests and needs.

For those working in agriculture, consider that your produce is god-given. By obeying the teachings garnered from nature; through observation of the leaf and root conditions and responding with due care, the result will be a good harvest. An example is adjusting the amount of water or fertiliser.

Follow the heart and think positively

Generally, animals and plants have a natural affinity to gather at bright, sunlit places or pleasant areas.

When a potted plant is placed by a window, veins and leaves grow towards the exposed light.

At a hotel I visited in Taiwan, all the flowers and leaves in the large floor pots were facing not towards the hotel guests, but towards the sun's brightness. Insects are attracted to buzz around streetlights at night. Cats like to lie in the warm sunlight.

To reiterate, to head for the bright spots or the pleasant places is a natural instinct of animals and plants. On the other hand, people will endure hardship and difficult circumstances, thinking that situations will eventually turn for the better. It is however, rather unnatural to behave in this manner. The heart will be eased if things are done that engender feelings of comfort.

Nevertheless, it is difficult to feel comfortable all the time, like when we have both good and bad health conditions. Often times we experience happiness when everything comes in our favour. At other times, we experience a negative or sad time with such things as losing a job, failing in a business or emotional heartbreak. Even in a difficult time, it is necessary to keep dynamic positive thinking to avoid depression.

It is no use to grumble to other people. People listening do not feel nice from the negativity, even if they show their sympathy, and after all, they will not be able to re-establish a lost business or bring a broken relationship back.

Instead of expressing regret for the past, people around will eagerly offer support when talking and acting positively; in the vein of, "I would like to do….. in my next job", or," I would like to associate with… type of person… in my next relationship",

It is human to admit a failure (even I have had many failures) and to think positively about the next step on the day after can be hard. The body can become stiffer under such unhealthy mental conditions.

With hope, the mind will open, life seems brighter and the body becomes softer.

Breaking boundaries creates an open heart

To open the mind, it is necessary to search out and eliminate 'pride and armouring', which maintains our outward appearances. Due to titles and work hierarchy, some people become irritated when they are unable to consider different outlooks and ideas from others, particularly when dissimilar from their own views. If such people are able to correct their attitude by listening to others openly and respond back to them along the lines of, "Right, my suggestion was inappropriate. Let's consider yours instead", they would feel respite and more comfortable in their communication with others.

It is the same at home.

There may be feelings of irritation by an opposed opinion from children and/or partner. However, a frank apology to them when a mistake is realised regardless of personal position would be more agreeable.

It's better to think akin to, "By apologising to them, not only they, but I also, feel better".

By overriding one's own stubbornness, which makes not only surrounding people but also oneself feel uncomfortable, the rigid heart will soften.

Nevertheless, there are some cases where people had best keep some stubbornness. Do insist on being tenacious for things considered fun, that create comfort and hope. Please, be obstinate with positive thinking to make your dreams come true! Examples would be: studying a foreign language for an overseas visit, improving skills in a sport, goal setting etc.

Finding the cause of prejudice offers clues to open the heart

When mentally suffering, it is important to think about the source, not only from a personal point of view, but also from different angles. For distress at work, think about it from the perspectives of the boss, a co-worker, a junior worker, and write down any conclusions. This helps to find the source of what or where an attitude or concept is actually being harboured.

HOGUSHI Massage helps to identify a cause of pain; then provides release and removal of the physical effects of that for the physical body. The process of releasing the mind is the same. After finding the cause of the pain by reflective contemplation from various angles, the next step is to get rid of it and release the mind's hold.

'What are the traps of this current cycle that are causing this pain?' Analyse the emotions and consider the ways to make people around you and yourself feel better.

Animals and plants have such a mind. It is known that vegetables grow healthy and cows produce quality milk with classical music played around them, thus creating a positive environment. Human beings have a mind with animal instincts, as well as the primal emotions.

The environment after birth influences the emotions

When people observe the exact same phenomena, some can consider it beautiful, and others may not. Even with children born of the same family, siblings will not have the same emotions or character as the life situations and times they were born into were different. Humans' emotions are formed by the various influences from parents, siblings, teachers, media and the people around us.

In the Lotus Sutra, it is said, "sarva-dharma-anaatman", which means- 'people are influenced by many people, though they seem to live freely by themselves'.

To illustrate, young children are influenced by their parents' tastes and habits, such as an addiction like gambling which is a negative role model.

A child may develop a negative complex from a reprimand by a teacher, or overconfidence from exuberant praise.

Realising that the cause of mental pain is actually an emotional memory and knowing where this emotion comes from, enables you to better comprehend the state of mind. Further reflection could be similar to; "I am currently suppressing this …counter opinion… because I feel this …complex… from previous experience", and then being able to control the behavioural response and improve the mental state.

Though you wish, you are unable to change others. If you are able to change your own way of thinking, you feel better and this has a positive effect on those around you. Don't be stubborn with an outlook like, "once decided there is no room for change". One way to improve things is by being unequivocally open to others to encompass a fair judgement, which then provides mental release through understanding and communication. As the ways of feeling are unlimited, it is important for you to be as creative as possible to make both yourself and others feel comfortable.

Three principles to open your heart

The methods to open the mind have already been mentioned in this chapter. Here I summarise them in three rules.

> **1. Knowing the reason (The Lotus Sutra)**
> **2. Being open minded (The Heart Sutra)**
> **3. Changing the way of thinking (The Lotus Sutra, Ch 25)**

The rigid mind is stubborn, always insisting on one's own opinion, judgement and experiences. Additionally, it automatically follows general consensus views, well-known theories and word from authority. It is not being open to others or considering other's positions. To release this rigidity of mind, it is important to follow the three rules.

The meaning of No.1, "Knowing the reason", is to know the cause of a difficulty with others.

People with a rigid mind often have troubles with others and it is important for these people to become aware of their inflexible mind and try to discover the reason for it.

Bad movements in sports, incorrect attitudes at work and poor diet will all contribute to developing some diseases or injuries through physical inflexibility. A narrow way of thinking also contributes to an inflexible mind.

By knowing the reason of how a habit of mind has developed, who has influenced this and why the thinking is thus, it is possible to correct the conceptual belief. Additionally, understanding the reasoning of others can allow one to forgive.

The meaning of No.2, "Being open minded" is to not insist on opinions based on consensus, popular theories and subjective positional views. Don't bother with small and petty things from others' point of view. The stubborn mind responds with suffering when complaints from others 'hit a nerve' or complex. We are released from pain when the effects of thinking beliefs are dissipated and an open mind attitude is sought.

The meaning of No.3, "Change the way of thinking" is to think of things from others' point of view. It is normal that everyone has his or her own way of thinking and feeling.

It puts one in an unpleasant position if there is anger and emotion when others do not agree with an expressed viewpoint. Such stubbornness can provide constant trouble with others. When things do not go the way wanted, keep in mind to change the way of thinking, for both yourself and others, to feel comfortable.

Ideal heart condition:

Steady mind – Let it move like a willow tree and flow like water

"Imperturbability" does not mean "Unmoving mind" at all. "Unmoving mind" is the same condition as "Dead mind". "Imperturbability" is actually the perpetually moving mind, which always provides the sense of, 'who', I am.

For example, willow trees always move in response to any wind. When the wind stops, they return to the position where they were in repose.

Water can fit in a container regardless of shape; it changes its form to ice when frozen and steam when boiled, but water is still water, itself.

When it comes to food, Tofu is a good example. It absorbs various other flavours within it, such as in; Sukiyaki, Mapo Doufu, Hot Pot as well as Hiyayakko (Chilled Tofu), but the flavour of Tofu itself never changes.

In other words, "Imperturbability" means to be in the condition of an extremely flexible mind without losing yourself. Under this circumstance of "Imperturbability", you won't be trapped with an inflexible mind and body.

The more flexible the body, the more open the heart

It has been mentioned before, that once the mind is eased, the body also becomes softer. The counter condition is also the same, once the body is softer with HOGUSHI Massage and stretching, it is easier to release the mind.

When the body is more flexible the breathing patterns become deeper and a feeling of relaxation is evident as the oxygen spreads throughout the body. It is like the feeling of relaxation from having a bath due to better blood flow and relieved muscles.

When the body is inflexible in a difficult situation, or abused, the mind and body respond instantly by becoming rigid.

On the other hand, if you maintain a softer body by applying HOGUSHI Massage and stretching regularly, you are able to stay calm even in difficult situations, similar to, "Well, it does not matter... though there was abuse" or "What was said might be true and I might have said something wrong to them".

When the body is relaxed we can still manage to think positively, even under stress.

I would like all of you to have a physically and mentally healthy life through releasing the body and the mind.

Voices from Participants

It's great that I'm able to maintain my body using HOGUSHI Massage by myself no matter how tired I am.

~ Ms Kiyomi Murakami in her 20's in Fukushima prefecture

There was a yoga and pilates boom at the time I studied fitness and aerobics and I also practised jazz and hip hop dance. Though still young at the time, I began yoga as I thought it would be good for maintaining my over-used body.

I found Family Yoga four years ago and took the general classes. I then studied the teachers' training course and joined the trips to Taiwan and Australia after the completion of my course. Currently, I run yoga classes in my hometown, Koriyama.

Until the time I learnt HOGUSHI Massage at Family Yoga, I had no idea of how to release the body after hard use. Although I've been building and stretching muscles, I had the idea that to release the body I had to visit acupuncturists or osteopaths.

I sensed that my body was becoming softer after HOGUSHI Massage on my hips at classes.

I'm pleased as I master HOGUSHI Massage to be able to maintain my body myself, no matter how tired I am. I've also had the sense and understanding that the softer my body became, the more my mind has opened.

At my classes, I use HOGUSHI Massage (which is Family Yoga's unique method), and my students say, "it's really good". There was a person who was unable to release their lower back pain at all, even with Tai Chi and aerobics. They were able to get rid of the pain after applying HOGUSHI Massage at my yoga class after only three times.

I feel that HOGUSHI Massage is not just a massage method; but provides us with something excellent as a total body response.

During my first training trip to Australia, some participants were sceptical when Mr and Mrs Ishii taught HOGUSHI Massage at a workshop, but during my second training trip they were actually practising it as they had seen how good it was.

Though diet and body structures differ from each other, I realised HOGUSHI Massage is effective regardless of background.

I suffered from persistent lower back pain due to my work for decades. I got rid of it by doing HOGUSHI Massage and stretching just once a week.

~ Mr Akira Hasegawa in his 60's in Tokyo prefecture

As I've been working as a taxi driver, I sit in the car everyday for a long time. I'd been suffering from lower back pain and stiff shoulders for decades, so I regularly had massage and visited the sauna which helped to release the pain for a while, but not permanently.

Three years ago, my daughter who regularly attended yoga classes at Family Yoga suggested I should join the class, so I tried taking the class once a week. By applying HOGUSHI Massage on my hips and practising yoga poses with guidance from the teachers, my pain in the lower back and the shoulders vanished and I no longer need to see my masseur. It removes tiredness and stress and makes me feel relaxed.

It's much better to maintain my body by myself as the effect seems to last longer and I don't have to rely on someone else.

Additionally, by doing the various yoga poses, the muscles, which I normally don't use, are stimulated and my body balance is maintained. I don't catch a cold now.

I felt uncomfortable at the first visit because only a few male participants were there at the classes, but I became a regular member, as my condition improved as long as I regularly took the class.

I would like to continue my work as long as possible with maintenance of my health by HOGUSHI Massage and yoga poses.

While still practising yoga at Family Yoga I have also been teaching twice a week at a nursing ward institution for 3 years. My students are mainly people who drop their family members at the day care centre. As they usually support their family members at home, they tend to have lower back pain and stiff shoulders, so I mainly focus on teaching hip work to release them.

In the beginning, I taught them Hips HOGUSHI Massage, such as rocking the areas in the stretched leg seated position, with arms behind the body. As the class space is so big, I also taught them "Hip walking" which is moving forward using hip muscles while keeping the same seated position, while raising the arms vertically to the sky.

They said it was difficult to move with raised arms, so I modified the pose to just raising the arms slightly, which looked like a dance, the 'Awaodori', one of the traditional Japanese dances, and they enjoyed it with many smiles.

I'm surprised that even though all the students in my class are over 70 years old, they gradually became flexible, have developed healthy facial colour and become more expressive.

Particularly a lady in her 80's who has pain in her knees. She achieved sitting on the heels (seiza) and was so pleased when other members told her she looked in her 20's from behind.

I was taught that the body becomes softer when the mind is opened. Though I did not understand the meaning of it when I was student, I really came to understand it when I became a teacher, especially when I witnessed that even aged people were still able to soften their body with a positive mind.

With the growing aged society, I sense that HOGUSHI Massage will be effective to make our life, physically and mentally healthy. So, I'd like to teach HOGUSHI Massage to as many people as possible.

Even though I was only able to reach 20cm above the ground in Standing Forward Bend, my palms can now reach the ground!

~ Ms M T In her 30's in Tokyo prefecture

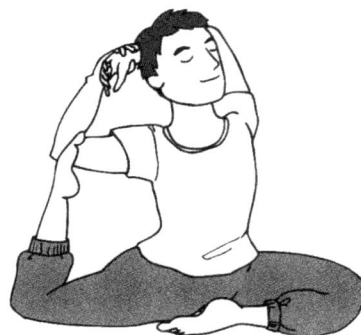

I started yoga five years ago at Family Yoga as I suffered from cramps; sensitivity to cold and a stiff body due to daily desk work in the design industry.

Though I couldn't sense the benefit of HOGUSHI Massage at the beginning, I was gradually able to feel that my body was softening, and even now do Hips HOGUSHI Massage at home every day because I feel awkward without it.

Due to my stiff body, I was initially only able to reach 20cm above the ground in Standing Forward Bend. It gradually became softer and now my palms reach the ground.

I also realise the level of cramping has reduced in the months I've been practising. I sense that yoga and HOGUSHI Massage are effective as the pain comes back when I cannot attend yoga sessions regularly due to work commitments during busy times.

I'm now able to be sensitive to the cold and when I recognise it in the early stages, I can deal with it by warming the area before it gets worse.

Due to yoga and HOGUSHI Massage, I think I've learnt how to sense the condition of my body successfully.

I apply HOGUSHI Massage before playing soccer. It makes me feel lighter and gives me better mobility.

- Mr Masahiko Yukawa in his 50's in Tokyo prefecture

I've been crazy about soccer since I was in junior high school and even now I still play it during weekends.

I have been a member of Family Yoga for 16 years and in the class we apply HOGUSHI Massage to the whole body, from the tip of the toes to the top of the head.

I always do HOGUSHI Massage before playing soccer.

As the muscles and joints are released, it makes me feel light and gives me better mobility.

I think it also helps me to prevent injuries such as sprains.

After playing soccer, the muscles and joints are stiffer due to hard use but applying HOGUSHI Massage reduces the fatigue and stiffness.

As I'm getting older, stamina and skills tend to decay. Though I'm 55 years old now, I feel the speed of decay is slower compared with my 30's. I consider it's due to yoga asanas and HOGUSHI Massage.

Practising Karate after HOGUSHI Massage,
the legs are solidly grounded and it makes me stand firm.
~ Ms Kyoko Kawase in her 30's in Tokyo prefecture

I've been practising Karate since I was in the second year primary school. As my Karate teacher was a good friend of the Family Yoga teacher, Mr Ishii, I also attended yoga classes for six months.

I thought I was flexible as I was able to open my legs easily in the Karate practice, however, I realised that I was wrong because I was unable to follow advanced levels of HOGUSHI Massage. The parts of the body used frequently in Karate such as the shoulders, torso, sides, calves and ankles were surprisingly stiff.

Mr Ishii taught me how to release particular parts and muscles with HOGUSHI Massage and my body gradually became softer.

I took the yoga teachers' course at Family Yoga a year ago, because I have a dream to be a Karate teacher in the future and I'd like to teach my students not only Karate but also HOGUSHI Massage.

I practise and introduce HOGUSHI Massage to my Karate friends to release the toes and the ankles. It has gathered a very good reputation as they have similar feelings as I have, like being able to feel they are standing firm and well grounded.

Tanden and Ki

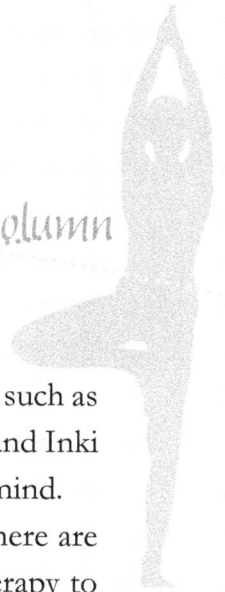

Although Ki is not yet scientifically proven, there are many related words in Japanese such as Genki (Energy/Spirit), Yaruki (Motivation), Youki (Cheerfulness), Byouki (Illness), and Inki (Melancholy). These are intangible concepts, but have influences on our body and mind.

In Oriental Medicine, the existence of Ki is a prerequisite. It is thought that there are paths (meridians) in our body through which Ki travels. Thus, acupuncture is a therapy to make Ki move within the body by stimulating the tsubo (the specific acupuncture points).

Yoga focuses on taking not only oxygen but Ki (Prana) into the body by breathing. Ki is important because it is enriching.

Ki in the body is centred at Tanden (the point below the navel). The Tanden is not an organ and it is thought of as a place where Ki is gathered. When Ki is held in Tanden the upper body is relaxed as the body weight has sunk lower; the mind is relaxed and the body becomes stable.

The Japanese phrase "Fundoshi wo shimenaosu" means to "Re-tighten the loincloth". To explain - the place where the knot of the loincloth is made with the tie-string is Tanden. The expression means that the people gathered Ki in the Tanden, relaxed their minds, enhanced their energy (when tired) and got themselves ready to accomplish something.

On the other hand, when Ki goes up above the Tanden the mind can become dizzy and feel uncomfortable. Physically, there may be pain felt in the pit of stomach or around the stomach and the pelvis does not tuck in.

By gathering Ki in Tanden, the posture naturally corrects, such as chin tucked in, chest open, pelvis tucked in and elbows squeezed towards the body.

Tanden helps you to be in balanced alignment with less fatigue.

Try to focus on gathering Ki in Tanden on a daily basis.

By maintaining correct posture in sports and movement we are able to prevent injuries and enjoy sport and competition with a relaxed mind.

www.ingramcontent.com/pod-product-compliance
Lightning Source LLC
Chambersburg PA
CBHW081159270326
41930CB00014B/3217